WHISTLE BLOWING
AND ETHICS IN HEALTH AND SOCIAL CARE

ANGIE ASH

Jessica Kingsley *Publishers*
London and Philadelphia

First published in 2016
by Jessica Kingsley Publishers
73 Collier Street
London N1 9BE, UK
and
400 Market Street, Suite 400
Philadelphia, PA 19106, USA

www.jkp.com

Library of Congress Cataloging in Publication Data
A CIP catalog record for this book is available from the Library of Congress

British Library Cataloguing in Publication Data
A CIP catalogue record for this book is available from the British Library

ISBN 978 1 84905 632 8
eISBN 978 1 78450 108 2

Printed and bound in Great Britain

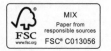

MIX
Paper from
responsible sources
FSC® C013056

This book is dedicated to the men and women who speak out about corruption, wrongdoing and injustice, and to those who stand by them when they do.

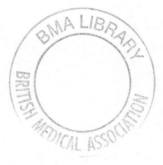

ACKNOWLEDGEMENTS

I am grateful to colleagues and scholars who generously supplied me with some of their work: Professor Guy B. Adams, University of Missouri; Professor Janet Near, Indiana University; Dr Joseph A. Petrick, Wright State University; Professor Linda K. Treviño, The Pennsylvania State University.

Professor David Lewis of Middlesex University kindly helped me understand a little better provisions of the UK's 1998 Public Interest Disclosure Act. Remaining legal blunders are entirely mine.

Fi Powell and Monmouthshire County Council libraries and information services always went the extra mile to locate material and provide information for me. They provide a truly outstanding public service.

And finally my warm thanks and great appreciation to Barrie for standing by my writing about speaking out, with all that was entailed along the way.

CONTENTS

ABBREVIATIONS

NGO Non-governmental organization, such as a charity or not-for profit agency
NHS National Health Service (UK)
PCaW Public Concern at Work, a UK whistleblowing NGO
PIDA Public Interest Disclosure Act 1998 (UK)

CHAPTER 1

THE PARADOX OF WHISTLEBLOWING

Many who report wrongdoing in the workplace – whistleblowers – become targets of harassment, intimidation, investigation, persecution and prosecution, to name but some acts of retaliation. The whistleblower may well be protected in law in a number of jurisdictions globally (the UK is one), yet that protection may not save them from the personal damage and professional detriment that is losing their job, career, family and financial security.

Great claims are often heard about the heroism of whistleblowing and whistleblowers. Public Concern at Work (PCaW), a UK whistleblowing charity, paid tribute to the 'important role that whistleblowing plays in achieving effective governance and an open culture', and regarded whistleblowing as 'one of the most effective ways to uncover fraud against organisations' (PCaW 2013, p.5). Fine words may pour forth from the mouths of politicians, usually long after the mobilization of state-funded retaliation against the whistleblower has done its work. The then UK Prime Minister, David Cameron, said in the House of Commons in answer to an oral question on 24 April 2013 that, '…we should support whistleblowers and what they do to help improve the provision of public services'. While it's always nice to be appreciated, even by a prime minister, the damage and destruction meted out to the whistleblower after they put their head above the parapet to speak out, suggests that relying on any appreciative accolades would be ill-advised. Grand words about the great job the whistleblower may do sit uneasily alongside evidence of the collateral, lifelong damage to lives, livelihoods, relationships, careers and health of those who stepped up to speak out: the whistleblowers.

PATTERNS OF PARADOX

Whistleblowing is the raising of a concern in the workplace or externally, about malpractice, poor practice, wrongdoing, risk or danger that affects others. There is no common definition of whistleblowing internationally. The whistleblower is a person who raises concerns in the public interest. They may not recognize themselves as such at the time they do this. Their concerns may be about the safety of a patient or user of health or social care services, or the integrity of the health or care system itself, as in the case of theft, waste, deception and duplicity (Francis 2015).

Whistleblowing – the act, the response, as well as the deafening silence of those who stand by in the face of wrongdoing – touches some very deep recesses of what it is to be human, to bear witness to wrongdoing, or to turn away. Most employees have observed wrongdoing. But most employers do not act to stop wrongdoing they know is going on (Miceli, Near and Dworkin 2009). These are but some of the paradoxes that whistleblowing presents, and which this book examines.

The UK prime minister quoted above was barely out of college when Stephen Bolsin took up post as a consultant anaesthetist at the Bristol Royal Infirmary (BRI) in England in 1988. From the start of his time in that hospital, Stephen Bolsin was troubled by the very high mortality rates for children undergoing heart surgery. Bolsin's were very serious concerns, substantiated by data on mortality outcomes. He raised these matters repeatedly with senior consultants in the hospital, with the national Department of Health, and the General Medical Council, the UK regulatory body of registered medical practitioners. When no action was taken by the hospital or the Department of Health, Bolsin took his concerns to the media. This prompted inquiry by the General Medical Council. Dr Bolsin was struck off the medical register. In 1995, he left the UK to work in Australia. Nineteen years after Bolsin first raised concerns, the public inquiry chaired by Ian Kennedy concluded that between 30 and 35 children had died unnecessarily, and that one-third of children undergoing heart surgery at the BRI prior to 1995 had had less than adequate care. The Kennedy Inquiry found Dr Bolsin had been right to persist in raising his concerns. It recommended a new culture of openness within the National Health Service (NHS), with a non-punitive system for reporting serious incidents (Hammond and Bousfield 2011; Kennedy 2001).

Fourteen years after Kennedy reported, the public inquiry chaired by Robert Francis into the failures of care in Mid Staffordshire NHS Foundation Trust reached that very same conclusion: the need for a culture of openness in the NHS. (Francis 2013a, b, c). A few months after Robert Francis reported in 2013, Dr Bolsin was awarded the Royal College of Anaesthetists' Medal in recognition of his work to promote safety in anaesthesia (PCaW 2013). Such is whistleblowing's pattern of paradox: blame the messenger for the message and hammer them hard. Then, after significant life-ending failures of care, spend millions of public money on public inquiries which, after several years, conclude that both messenger and message had been pretty much right all along.

THE WHISTLEBLOWER'S PROTECTION

The Public Interest Disclosure Act 1998 (PIDA) went onto the UK statute book some years after Dr Bolsin had raised concerns about child mortality rates, been struck off the medical register and relocated to another continent. The UK was one of the first EU states to legislate to protect whistleblowers. PIDA is intended to provide protection to people who make protected disclosures. Yet, in another paradox, the experience of people who blow the whistle on poor, corrupt and unethical practice, is seldom anything other than negative. Witnessing what happens to whistleblowers does not inspire others to do likewise, the House of Commons Health Committee concluded in 2014 (HOC 2014).

The use of so-called 'gagging orders' in the NHS was another twist in the tail of whistleblower protection. Payment of these gags in the UK NHS was halted in 2013, meaning special payments made outside an employee's contract have to make clear that nothing in such an agreement prevents the individual whistleblowing in the future.

That these gagging orders existed at all was denied in 2013 by the then Chief Executive of NHS England, David Nicholson (Ramesh 2013). Nicholson claimed some people *felt* they'd been gagged'; and that the case of the whistleblower contacted by NHS lawyers, who threatened to demand repayment of their settlement agreement if they spoke out, 'was a mistake' (Aitkenhead 2013). Be that as it may, a request made by a Member of Parliament under UK Freedom of Information legislation revealed that the NHS had spent over £2m on over 50 'gagging orders' between 2008 and 2013 (Hughes 2013).

Nicholson's denial that gagging orders existed (it is important to notice the syntactical sleight where people are said to *feel* gags existed) was news to Gary Walker, who had been sacked as chief executive from United Lincolnshire Hospitals Trust in 2010 (Walker 2015). As chief executive, Walker had raised patient safety concerns about hospital capacity to meet government targets for non-emergency care. Walker was later dismissed for allegedly swearing in a meeting, an allegation he denied and said a witness statement disproved. Walker intended to present that statement, and other evidence, to the scheduled 15-day employment tribunal hearing in 2011. On the first day of this tribunal, his NHS employers offered Walker £320,000 to settle the claim. With legal fees, Walker estimated the NHS spent over £500,000 getting rid of him. This seems a remarkable sum of public cash to fork out if there were no patient safety concerns. It would be a truly incredible amount to pay to silence someone alleged to have sworn in a meeting. When, in 2013, Walker went public about his patient safety concerns, he was threatened with legal action by his erstwhile NHS employers. That would seem, *prima facie*, a threat to silence – or, in the vernacular, a gag.

LIVING WITH PARADOX

The paradox of whistleblowing stretches much wider yet than a semantic 'gag' or 'no gag'. From outside health and social care services, say from the perspective of the patient or user of one of those services, speaking out about bad practice or mistreatment of adults or children vulnerable through sickness or circumstance, is a no-brainer. Why would a trained professional, or any concerned observer, *not* raise their concerns? But then, when they do, why are there so few whistleblowers who, unequivocally, say they are glad they broke ranks to speak out, and that their disclosures were an excellent career move that they commend to others?

These paradoxes show up in UK public attitudes towards whistleblowing, and use of the term itself. A British survey of 2000 people found eight in ten believed it was more important to support, and not punish, people who blew the whistle. But fewer than half (47 per cent) thought British society found whistleblowing generally acceptable, or that managers were serious about protecting whistleblowers (Vandekerckhove 2012). Inevitably, and reflecting these conflicted attitudes, the word 'whistleblowing' itself attracts a negative valence, with the anodyne 'raising concerns' suggested as a preferable substitute to use with employees (OPCW 2012). Changing a word is one way of ducking the paradoxes. Another is to look at those conflicted contradictions head-on, and wonder what it is we do to people, organizations and health and social care, when we can't name what is going on before us.

Individual and public reaction to whistleblowing and to the whistleblower are, then, riddled with paradox. These paradoxes conflict us all, whether whistleblower, bystander, or victim of wrongdoing. Culturally, certainly in the UK and the western world, the rugged individualist is venerated; but then of course we love the team player. Social pressures to fit in, coexist with those pushing us to stand out. The workplace demands that employees do things right; the public wants people who'll do the right thing. Whistleblowers may be the butt of retaliation; yet their retaliators escape scrutiny. News, film, culture, love the lone ranger, yet loathe the oddball who wonders out loud if the emperor really is wearing any clothes. The whistleblower is feted, yet crushed; hailed as a hero, punished as a scapegoat.

SPEAKING OUT AS NOT BEING HEARD

Public reaction to the caricature of 'care' provided in some parts of the Mid Staffordshire NHS Foundation Trust in England between 2005 and 2009 was shock, dismay, distress. Yet many people working in those very services had raised concerns, only to find themselves ignored, marginalized, ostracized or scapegoated. Most simply gave up trying to get anything changed (Francis 2013a). In the face of this, few could take issue with the House of Commons Health Committee which, in its report on complaints and raising concerns in the NHS, said a 'means must be found for health and care service workers to be able to speak up safely about professional concerns'. Still less, that 'there is an unambiguous professional duty on professional registrants to speak up, but that equally there is a similar duty on employers to establish an open culture which encourages concerns to be raised and acts to address and resolve them, rather than punish the person raising them' (HOC 2015, p.35). This Committee concluded that the detriment so many whistleblowers suffer has undermined public trust in the system's ability to treat whistleblowers with fairness and, crucially (as if that were not enough), that this lack of confidence had implications for patient and citizen safety.

The paradox of all this is that whistleblowing is an act of loyalty, a commitment to doing right, to doing no more harm. That is prosocial behaviour, not deviance. The whistleblower's 'crime' is their acting against the code of silence – that organizational *omertà* – which is, in dysfunctional organizational cultures, inexplicably conflated with loyalty. They may be vilified, typecast as a rat, snitch or 'difficult'; as mentally ill, malicious or vengeful. (The particular slant of denigration varies.) Or, conversely, once the wrongdoing has been exposed to public opprobrium, they may enjoy 15 minutes of fame and be celebrated as a hero, before they turn to face the toll that speaking out has exacted on their future career prospects, personal relationships, and any possibility of financial security in what remains of their lives.

The more systematic the wrongdoing, the greater the reprisal. Speak out about wrongdoing that is widespread – the 'new normal' of the organization, say – and which involves a lot of cash, then those reprisals are likely to be whistleblower-crushing. Most whistleblowers don't work in their employment field again. Some lose their homes, profession and health, to depression, alcoholism, family break-up. Still more, the greatest shock to the whistleblower is likely to be what they learn about the world in its reaction to their speaking out (Alford 2001).

These paradoxes lie at the heart of whistleblowing and they affect us all. That rugged, autonomous individual, so beloved of media or marketers, is quashed when the organization mobilizes its 'vast resources in the service of the individual's destruction' (Alford 2001, pp.3–4). Alford, a psychoanalyst and political scientist, suggested we listen to that individual – the whistleblower – so that 'we may learn something, not just about individuality, but about the forces that confront it' (Alford 2001, p.4). This book sets out to contribute to that learning.

WHAT THIS BOOK IS ABOUT

This book starts from 'the point' (in both senses) of these paradoxes, that is, their location and their meaning. Its premiss is this: unless and until we wake up and face in to see these paradoxes at play in responses to whistleblowing, then the familiar, formulaic responses to shocking failures in health and social care – expensive public inquiries years after the event; retribution and silencing of those who spoke out, 'tightening up' of standards and targets that missed the point first time round, to name but some – will fail those who use those services, and those who speak out about problems in them. The irreplaceable public goods that are publicly-funded health and social care services are simply too precious to allow a systemic wilful blindness to these paradoxes, and their consequences, to prevail. Shining a light on those and on their systemic backcloth is what the whistleblower does and, in so doing, pays the price. Maybe it's time for those who are elected to serve, lead, regulate and run those organizations to look, listen, and share that load a little.

Three distinct strands give shape to the book's architecture. First is the significance of organizational culture and leadership in shaping the possibility that people will step up to speak out about poor practice. Organizational culture and its leadership (and that includes its political, policy and regulatory dimensions) can make or break the likelihood of whistleblowing, with or without further duties to report wrongdoing being imposed on professionals. Leadership (its style, culture and manner that are imprinted throughout the organization), and organizational culture, are interdependent, and – for better or for worse – overwhelmingly powerful influences on what happens in organizations, and to the whistleblower.

Organizational culture, with its norms, values, beliefs and behaviours is a dynamic, fluid, social construction. At any moment, people act in line with social norms, conventions and expectations (Warren 2003). The dynamics of working in teams – their power relations, group pressures to conform, to fit in, be a good team player – receive passing attention, at best, in a drive to pin blame on 'someone', occasionally on 'something', when things go wrong. Well-established findings on, for example, bystanders (why do people ignore somebody in pain?), silence (why do people keep quiet in the face of wrongdoing?), punishment (why do otherwise well-adjusted human beings inflict suffering on others when an authority tells them to do so?) and administrative evil (why do people not recognize that the bit part they may play in organizational life may contribute to larger destructive consequences?) receive little explicit attention. What are these saying about the organization's response to the whistleblower or to the concerns they raise?

In his independent review into creating an open and honest reporting culture in the NHS, *Freedom to Speak Up*, Robert Francis concluded that there was a need for culture change in the NHS (Francis 2015). Francis disaggregated various domains of culture as follows. Safety was first; then a culture of raising concerns; one free from bullying; a culture with visible leadership and one of valuing staff; and finally, a culture of reflective practice. This book upends that order; it puts reflective practice first. Without that, we cannot realize the others. Without reflective practice that fronts ethical and moral action (to provide best possible care and to speak out about shortcomings), we cannot ensure patient and user safety. There can be little value to visible leadership unless it reflects, models, expects, lives and breathes ethical health or social care. Without reflection – going beyond the superficial – we will not understand, still less tackle, bullying, the abuse of power, scapegoating and the other mucky stuff that whistleblowing throws up. Without reflection – staring out some some blunt truths about how relationships of power, authority and obedience play out in organizational life – any chance of realizing a brave new world where people speak out as a matter of routine about shortcomings of health and care will remain remote.

The book's second strand argues that, at its core, the act of whistleblowing is a moral activity. It has moral consequences, for good or bad, for the person raising concerns, and the person(s) or practice(s) those concerns are raised about. Yet the ethics and morality of whistleblowing, or of practices and behaviours and what goes on in the workplace, are seldom construed as such. The concept of 'morality' doesn't play out well in political, public and professional discourse that is hell-bent on reducing genuine understanding of what went wrong and why, to reprisal, retaliation and retribution, as well as production of the obligatory action plan with accompanying statements that lessons have been learned. It's too academic, too vague, too well-meaning to get the attention of the politician needing a headline. But the ethics of health and social care are the core, the basis, the means and the infrastructure of how we do our business together as people who need the care of others at points throughout our lives.

To give this traction, the book considers the four elements of an ethic of care – attentiveness, responsibility, competence, responsiveness – originally developed by Fisher and Tronto (1990). These four elements are used to propose an ethical structure that drives, imprints and manifests an ethic of care throughout health and social care delivery. This includes its leadership, management, policy-making and regulatory framework. Laying duties to deliver an ethic of care onto just one part of this structure – the individual delivering health or social care – will not ensure ethical care, without the wider health and social care system underwriting that duty, and supporting it explicitly, in word and deed.

Hence, and third, the book's focus and locus takes in, most certainly, the policy and regulatory system that frames the delivery of health and social care services. It is not a book about practice or practitioners, although failures of health and care find form there, at least superficially. The book, overtly and unequivocally, places the politics, policy and regulation of health and social care into analysis of the 'failure frame', and the response to whistleblowers who speak out. What happened in Mid Staffordshire NHS Foundation Trust was not a little local difficulty. It was cultural, systemic, and unambiguously implicated the social policy *zeitgeists* that surrounded, and corroded the delivery of decent healthcare to so many people.

Mostly UK focused, the book draws on learning, experiences and examples of whistleblowing internationally. Although it does not rehash disasters and scandals in health and social care (they come and go and will happen again if we continue to do what we do), three particular 'failures' of health and social care in England crop up from time to time throughout the book. These are the disasters that were the (now dissolved) Mid Staffordshire NHS Foundation Trust (then part of NHS England); Winterbourne View (a private healthcare assessment and treatment facility for people with learning disabilities); and the handling of systematic, prolonged, organized sexual exploitation of children and young people by Rotherham Metropolitan Borough Council and its partners. These three failures are discussed to pull out some common features of organizational responses to whistleblowing and the whistleblower: silence, denial, blame, retribution and turning those blind eyes and deaf ears.

CONUNDRUMS AND QUESTIONS

Overall, the book considers a number of conundrums and questions:

- What is whistleblowing, and why is 'whistleblowing' such a loaded word?

- Why don't people who are paid to lead, manage or provide professional or practical health and social care always raise concerns of poor or harmful practices when they encounter them?

- Why is demonstrably poor practice sometimes not 'seen', 'heard' or recognized as such in the workplace? Why the silence?

- What happens in the workplace, at the time and subsequently, to those who blow the whistle?

- What is organizational culture, and what part does it play in what goes on in the workplace, on right- and wrongdoing, and whistleblowing?

- What would ethical care, practice, policy, regulation, leadership and management look like in health and social care?

- How can ethical health and care systems be created, bedded in and sustained?

- How can 'raising concerns' become a routine, everyday, expected feature of how ethical health and care systems operate?

These questions are discussed throughout the book. Chapter 2 starts that discussion with an overview of whistleblowing, and what is known about the characteristics of whistleblowers. The protection afforded the whistleblower by UK whistleblowing legislation and policy is considered, as are acts of retaliation, retribution and their consequences for the whistleblower.

Chapter 3 moves the spotlight onto features and facets of organizational culture and, in particular, the whistleblower's action in bringing 'undiscussable' aspects of organizational life into the open. This chapter looks at how wrongdoing becomes normalized, rationalized and institutionalized in organizational culture. Individual moral agency of the individual versus the power of a group in shaping moral action are examined, as are the influences on speaking out or staying silent about wrongdoing. This chapter's elaborate metaphor mix – blind eyes and deaf ears abound in the company of bad apples, elephants in the room and the emperor's wearing of clothes – hints at the power of language both to contain and to name that which we are unwilling to face head on.

Chapter 4 continues this theme in its discussion of the 'shapes and sounds' of organizational silence and denial of wrongdoing. The propensity of ostensibly normal, well-adjusted people to inflict suffering on others when ordered to by authority is considered. The response of Rotherham Metropolitan Borough Council to the prolonged, systematic sexual exploitation of children and young people, over many years, is reviewed. Six 'devices of denial' used by the Council are identified to illustrate a systemic, institutionalized denial of harm.

Chapter 5 looks at the social phenomenon that is 'bystanding', or standing by and doing nothing when harm is perpetrated. Some of the complex features of self-deception involved in a tacit tolerance of poor, harmful or criminal practice are identified, including the human capacity to overestimate personal ethicality and morality.

In a change, if not a lightening, of tone, Chapter 6 discusses two commonly proffered remedies to encourage whistleblowing: paying people to speak up about wrongdoing, and laying a 'duty to whistleblow' on professionals. In light of the foregoing, these two 'remedies', often to be heard in post-disaster 'this must never happen again' pronouncements, are discounted. Ill-informed and simplistic, both fail to grasp the complexity, for the organization and people in it, present when the whistleblower steps up to speak out about poor health and social care.

Chapter 7, on whistleblowing and ethical health and social care systems, makes the case for an ethic of care to be imprinted *throughout* the health and social care system, including public policy, the regulation of health and social care and the organizations and services that employ health and social care professionals and others. The chapter maps out what this might mean, and how it might manifest. Its crux is the need for ethical care that, routinely and as a matter of course, is intolerant of poor, marginal or downright dangerous action, and which expects and encourages people to speak out.

Chapter 8 returns to the overwhelming significance of organizational culture, and of those in leadership positions, on the behaviour of people working in it. If an ethic of care is to drive the work of the health and social care system, and the speaking out about shortcomings of care, then it needs clear expression and realization by its leadership. The chapter considers what 'ethical' leadership would look like, how it would influence the organizational culture and its responses to whistleblowing. The emotional intelligence of the leader, their awareness of self, others, the culture and climate of the organization and its secrets and silence, are put forward as hallmarks of a leadership style that is well-positioned to deal, ethically, with disclosures a whistleblower makes.

Finally, Chapter 9 summarizes the critical need to understand whistleblowing as a moral act that requires a moral response. If the whistleblower is the messenger, why not listen?

WHAT THE BOOK IS NOT

This is a wake-up book, not a feel-good guide. That these things happen to whistleblowers should alert the reader, not render them mute, inert or silent. Nor is this a whistleblower's self-help manual, how-to handbook or legal sourcebook. There are good sources of help, and the book's Postscript on its final pages has a few words to say about these to a prospective whistleblower. These can be summarized: get wise and get prepared.

At some points, the author's weariness with the myopic policy fixation on delivering targets by any means necessary bleeds through. It would be wrong to read this as a call for targets, standards and the related regulatory apparatus to be junked. Not so. The problem isn't the targets or standards, but the obsession in hitting them, rather than understanding the point of them – the people, humanity, pain and suffering that lie behind the numbers. The problem is believing that targets, *ipso facto*, safeguard patients and citizens from harm. The problem is their deracination from an ethic of care and from the affective, human dimensions of competent health and caregiving. You may have been seen within two, four or however many hours the target for attention in Accident and Emergency is that day, but if you have a ruptured spleen and you are sent home with aspirin this (achieved) target says zilch about your health, care or prospects of survival.

There is not a great deal of evidence that training employees on ethics and morality has much resilience beyond the training room. In laying out these limitations, the book is not suggesting such training is worthless but that its application back at work is what counts. All that training has to be given the chance to work – in the workplace. If it's strangled at birth by a disinterested leadership who want the numbers of people trained but not the outcome, then the impact of this training will be negligible. It won't change a thing: what happens in the workplace will.

TERMS USED

Health and social care are used mostly as conjoined entities in this book, though the reality of health and social care service planning and provision in the UK is far from that. 'Health' is used to refer to regulated public or private healthcare. 'Social care' includes statutory or voluntary social work, provision of personal care, support to the person, whether adult or child. Aggregating adult and children's services in this way is done expeditiously. (In some parts of the UK adult and children's social services have been separated.) The point of the book is not the organizational structures of health and social care. They shift over time. Its concern is what happens inside those organizational entities when people speak out about wrongdoing. That changes much less.

Whistleblower and **person raising concerns**, and 'whistleblowing' and 'raising concerns' are used interchangeably, but legally they are different. The person *blowing the whistle*, if they are making a protected disclosure in law, has such protection as is afforded by whistleblowing legislation in place in their jurisdiction at the time of the disclosure.

CHAPTER 2

WHISTLEBLOWING

GOOD, BAD AND UGLY

Commentary, reaction, blame or praise about whistleblowing – take your pick – are not generally informed either conceptually or empirically. Whistleblowing can crop up in casual conversation when a whistleblower case hits the headlines. The general public may have a view, often of bewilderment, about the behaviour of those running the bank, corporation, health or social care organization that allowed the corruption, poor care or illegal activity to occur in the first place and, even more disconcertedly, of the retribution heaped on the whistleblower after their exposure of it. It is hard for the outside observer to grasp what appears to be the irrationality, if not insanity, of the denial/defence/blame response of large organizations to whistleblowers and the matters they raise concerns about. It seems to be even harder for those organizations to think more carefully about how they respond to the whistleblower.

This chapter provides an overview of whistleblowing, the whistleblower, and of what they may anticipate after they blow the whistle. First, some of the fables, fantasies and facts around whistleblowing and the public reaction to whistleblowers are discussed. Next, what whistleblowing is, both conceptually and practically, is considered, followed by, third, a review of the characteristics of whistleblowers. Fourth, what is involved for the whistleblower in weighing up the costs and benefits of speaking out is outlined, along with the double bind that is the requirement on the health or social care professional to report wrongdoing, and the detriment they personally may suffer when they do. The fifth part of the chapter, on UK whistleblowing legislation and policy, is a bridge (or breathing space) before the final section. This looks at what happens when people whistleblow, particularly the retaliation and retribution they may suffer, notwithstanding any protection under law they may have. Turning a blind eye to the possibility of retaliation is like turning away from the wrongdoing itself. Both are denial. Better for the whistleblower, and their managers, to face into this, than pretend it doesn't exist.

FABLES, FANTASIES AND FACTS

Media coverage of whistleblowing is fond of constructing a narrative of the lone hero taking on organizations, agencies, companies (as *Time* magazine's 2002 'Persons of the Year. The Whistleblowers' (Lacayo and Ripley 2002)) or sometimes an entire industry (such as the scientist Jeffrey Wigand's exposure of tobacco (Armenakis 2004)). This storyline plots the whistleblower's selfless drive to counter injustice and corruption, to stop harm and suffering being visited on people, animals, and the world in which we live, by the actions or inaction of organizations, corporations or professions. The 'selfless heroism' portrayal of the whistleblower and the whistleblowing dovetails nicely with the individualistic, 'small person against the big corporation', David v. Goliath cultural motif that sells front covers and makes blockbuster films. Goodies and baddies, heroes and villains, right and wrong, make good copy. It is a neat duality that has little or no concern with the lifelong, life-changing, personal, financial and human costs to the whistleblower and their family, or to the victimization, retaliation or ostracism they may well live with for the rest of their lives as a consequence of their raising concerns and speaking out.

In this vein, Grant (2002) wondered if whistleblowers were 'saints of secular culture'. Whether saint or sinner, the whistleblower and whistleblowing encapsulate conflicting and conflicted social values. We love the underdog taking on the organization, but hate sneaks, snitches and grasses. We revere the charismatic individualist, but at work want everyone to keep their head down, get on with their job and, above all, fit in with the team. There is public outrage about domestic violence, yet banging and shouts from next door are ignored and the TV turned up. We elevate 'family' and worship family life, but anyone speaking out about abuse and mistreatment by a family member had better watch out. Not seeing, not hearing and not speaking out about injustice coexist with relief that someone else did, and we're glad it wasn't us.

The popular narrative places great expectations on the whistleblowing act. The subtitle of Glazer and Glazer's (1989) book *The Whistleblowers* was *A New Tradition of Courageous Dissent.* Mansbach (2011) was of the view that whistleblowing protects the community, promotes the public good and extends the rule of law. Lewis, Brown and Moberly amplified this: '...whistleblowing is now established as one of the most important processes – if not *the* single most important process – by which governments and corporations are kept accountable to the societies they are meant to serve and service' (Lewis, Brown and Moberly 2014, p.1; emphasis in original). The accountability of huge corporations, industries and governments is, in a deft twist of logic, outsourced to the individual whistleblower, who also, of course, depends on that institution for their livelihood. The challenge that whistleblowing might once have presented to the company is thus co-opted and incorporated into huge organizations and governments, who then claim self-regulating 'social responsibility' (Pemberton *et al.* 2012).

WHAT WHISTLEBLOWING IS

Despite periodic media coverage, the social phenomenon that is 'whistleblowing' is underdeveloped both empirically and theoretically in the social sciences (Miceli and Near 2005; Pemberton *et al.* 2012). Internationally, and historically, most published studies and research have been carried out by US academics on US organizations (although that is now changing). Caution is needed before transferring lessons and learning from that economy and culture, with its particular approach to labour law, to other jurisdictions with very different legislation, legal protection, and approaches to employee rights protection in the workplace. There is a dearth of systematic analysis of the relationships between organizational characteristics that help whistleblowing: aggressive, neo-liberal, competitive and highly individualistic economies and economic frameworks such as in the US, are very different from the labour market and employment practices of, say, Norway (Pemberton *et al.* 2012; Skivenes and Trygstad 2010).

'Whistleblowing' itself is a US term, although it may have British origins in the practice of old-style police officers blowing a whistle if they suspected wrongdoing (Evans 2008). Whistleblowing is not complaining, suing or arguing. A whistleblower discloses information across a particular organizational boundary, whether internal (say, from one part of the organization to another) or external (from within the organization to the public domain) (Bouville 2008; Evans 2008). In the UK, whistleblowing in its legal sense is action taken by an employee under the Public Interest Disclosure Act 1998 (PIDA). Under this law, which is discussed below, a member of staff may assume protection against subsequent harassment or dismissal by employers when the employee makes a qualified disclosure of fraud or malpractice to a designated officer.

The commonly used definition of whistleblowing was set out by US academics Near and Miceli in the 1980s: '...the disclosure by organization members (former or current) of illegal, immoral or illegitimate practices under the control of their employers, to persons or organizations that may be able to effect action' (Near and Miceli 1985, p.4). Skivenes and Trygstad (2010) widened this to include all forms of communication where critical voices are raised about wrongdoing in the presence of someone who can stop the misconduct; and that includes day-to-day communication and critical discussions between managers and employees that are part of work, or should be. Skivenes and Trygstad regarded Near and Miceli's definition, above, as 'weak whistleblowing', or the first step taken when an employee raises concerns. They contrasted this with 'strong' whistleblowing, which 'focuses on *process* and on cases where there is no improvement in, or explanation for, or clarification of the reported misconduct from those who can do something about it' (Skivenes and Trygstad 2010, p.1077). In these cases, the employee has to report the matter again, hence Skivenes and Trygstad's notion of 'strong' whistleblowing, or turning up the volume on raising concerns, not giving up, and going outside the organization with the matter.

For Jubb (1999), six elements were necessary for the act of whistleblowing:

1. the act of disclosure itself

2. the person disclosing

3. the subject of the disclosure

4. the target of disclosure

5. the disclosure recipient

6. the outcome.

Jubb regarded whistleblowing, variously, as a public act of dissent, of conflicting loyalty, a deliberate non-obligatory act of disclosure. For the purposes of this book, 'whistleblowing' is used in its widest sense – that is, to describe acts of speaking out to raise concerns about the standard, legality and probity of practice in health and social care, and whether these matters are raised inside or outside the organization. These may be acts of dissent, as Jubb characterized whistleblowing. The act of whistleblowing may be about an organizational system, a process, or an entire sector, such as Wigand's disclosures on the tobacco industry in the US. Fundamentally however, whistleblowing (whether internal or external to the organization) has three defining features: first, intentional disclosure of information by an employee; second, the disclosure of concerns, malpractice or wrongdoing over which the organization has control or responsibility; and third, the purpose of the disclosure is to put right the malpractice or wrongdoing (Tsahuridu and Vandekerckhove 2008).

Whistleblowing itself is a *dynamic* process, in that the dynamics between the people involved and the particular situation interact when protected disclosures are made. This way of seeing whistleblowing assumes three (or more) parties: the person doing wrong, the person observing wrongdoing and the person who receives the report of wrongdoing (Near and Miceli 1996). This triad assumes the supposed wrongdoing is committed by an individual, rather than by some, or many, behaving and acting in accord with institutional practices, such as when corrupted health and caregiving become normalized, or systemic. Although whistleblowing gets personalized

– the individual whistleblower is named (and often shamed for their trouble) – the concerns they raise may be about bad, poor or dangerous practices that have become embedded, institutionally and structurally, in health and social care systems. The disaster of early twenty first-century healthcare in England at Mid Staffordshire NHS Foundation Trust was not that of a few isolated incidents, but systemic failures that many employees had tried to raise concerns about, and over a long period of time. Systematized bad practice – where workplace culture, ways of working or of treating people, becomes institutionalized and normalized – have been features of some of the worst health and social care scandals in the UK. Understanding this is critically important to prevent future harm, suffering, and sometimes death, being visited on sick or vulnerable people, and to recognize that those speaking out about harm are the organization's early warning system of failure.

WHO IS LIKELY TO WHISTLEBLOW AND ABOUT WHAT?

The sort of wrongdoing or bad practice that may lead to someone whistleblowing covers a wide spectrum. Your bad practice may be my self-justified corner-cutting to get the job done, please managers and hit targets. Brown (2008) pulled out six categories of wrongdoing from a large survey into public interest whistleblowing in Australian public sector agencies:

1. conflict of interest

2. improper or unprofessional behaviour

3. defective administration

4. waste or mismanagement of resources

5. perverting justice or accountability

6. personnel or workplace grievances.

This survey found whistleblowing to be more commonplace in the Australian public sector than had been expected; the most serious reported wrongdoings involved corruption, defective administration or waste.

As to who whistleblows, spotting personality traits and individual characteristics of the whistleblower doesn't provide a coherent picture of their profile. The search for the personality attributes, beliefs and motivations of whistleblowers yields a very mixed picture (Pemberton *et al.* 2012). Age is not a predictor of the propensity to whistleblow, but then employee age is usually inextricably bound up with other occupational variables, such as the employee's length of service, experience, nature of their tenure and supervisory status. Depending on the sector and industry, for example, older employees with security of tenure and more experience may be more likely to hold supervisory positions. In a review of the 2003 US National Business Ethics Survey, Stansbury and Victor (2009) found that individuals who were both young and with short organizational tenure were less likely to whistleblow. Again in the US, Near and Miceli (1996) found that whistleblowers were older, with longer tenure and higher educational attainment, than non-whistleblowing employees; they were thus more likely to be better paid and hold supervisory status that carried with it responsibility for rectifying wrongdoing. Employees who do not see whistleblowing as part of their job are less likely to raise a concern; those holding some scrutiny responsibilities in their place of work are more likely to report wrongdoing (Miceli and Near 2005). People with higher status and positional power in the organization tend to be more experienced and better paid, and generally to be more proactive in tackling problems and raising concerns (Miceli 2004). None of these findings is personality trait based. They are situational; that is, employees occupying a particular job in an organization, and having certain status and responsibilities to sort out problems, appear more likely to raise concerns.

The significant finding of Brown's Australian survey mentioned above, and others, is that with one exception there is little to distinguish whistleblowers from non-whistleblowers. You can hardly tell them apart on any of the usual matrices that differentiate employee competencies, skills and propensities. Whistleblowers hold the same attitudes about their workplace, about their job and about their managers as those who remained silent. Almost anybody in this survey could be expected to speak up and not – as retribution attacks by the organization on the whistleblower would have us believe – just those who were bitter, passed over for promotion or looking for a fight. By the same token, almost any employee could stay silent in the face of wrongdoing. Just one characteristic set those who spoke out apart from others, and that was the high level of 'organizational citizenship behaviour' they displayed – that is, they cared about the organization and took their role as part of it very seriously (Brown 2008).

So it is not simple to spot who will whistleblow. If an employer wanted to select (or deselect) people likely to speak out about wrongdoing, they could not easily pinpoint the killer qualities of the whistleblower. Attempts to identify individualized personality traits that set the whistleblower apart from their peers have generally been disappointing. Stansbury and Victor (2009) found that 'prosocial' behaviours (behaviour motivated by altruism as well as self-interest, and intended to benefit the public or social good), when reinforced and informally normalized in the workplace, were more likely to increase whistleblowing activity. Younger and short-tenured employees were less influenced by this prosocial control, suggesting that this is learned and reinforced over time in the workplace. As with the organizational citizenship behaviour found in Brown's (2008) study, when an employee displays prosocial behaviour – when they care about what they do and want to benefit the public or social good – they are more likely to raise concerns about practice. This prosocial behaviour needs an environment in which it is cultivated and valued: an organization and employer that is prosocial, and displays citizenship behaviour in what *it* does, and how it does it. Context counts.

The power of the context to influence whether employees speak out about concerns cuts both ways. Low-wage sectors and deregulated labour markets (as are significant parts of the US and UK economies), characterized by job insecurity and with limited, if any, employment protection, employing younger employees and women with young children, are more likely to be deterred from raising concerns (Zipparo 1999). Thus pre-existing structural inequalities impact on employee propensity to blow the whistle. Keeping children fed, warm and clothed while working antisocial hours in more than one minimum wage, zero hours job dampens down the appetite for upsetting the precarious applecart that is job (in)security. In health and social care services in the UK, care support workers are typically on minimum wage. The use of agency staff in health and social care services is widespread. These are not job conditions that encourage whistleblowing.

Even though they coined the term 'ethical resister', Glazer and Glazer (1989) agreed that the decision to report wrongdoing could not be attributed only to an individual's personal propensity to do so, or to any identifiable, innate features predisposing one person to raise concerns but not another. Jeff Wigand, the scientist who exposed the duplicity and corruption of the tobacco industry in concealing and misrepresenting data about smoking-related death rates, said there was no great epiphany for him when he went public with his concerns. Wigand came to regard what he did as an ethical decision, an incremental process of unsuccessfully raising concerns inside the organization, and then taking them outside the tobacco industry (Armenakis 2004).

There is, then, no clear profile of the 'typical' or 'predictable' whistleblower. Who whistleblows, why they do, why some chose one path and not the other, are not questions for which there are evidence-based answers (Bocchiaro, Zimbardo and Van Lange 2012). Searching for the individual traits and characteristics that constitute 'the whistleblower' overlooks the power and influence of the workplace context the whistleblower finds themselves in. Any search for individualized predictors of whistleblowing, devoid of attention to context, situation and power dynamics, is unlikely to produce anything other than a list of decontextualized, scientifically weak characteristics with little predictive or explanatory power. Personal and situational characteristics interact, but those contextual variables – the organization, its culture, relationships of power and authority, peer group pressures – explain the propensity to whistleblow more than individual factors (Near and Miceli 1996). If, for example, managers and supervisors routinely raise concerns (thus displaying prosocial organizational citizenship behaviour) the likelihood of a new employee doing so is greater, as they conform to the norms of the workplace and model their behaviour on more positionally powerful colleagues. Co-workers encourage or discourage whistleblowing through social reinforcement of workplace norms, and those informal structural characteristics of group behaviour tend to regulate member behaviour (Greenberger, Miceli and Cohen 1987). Thus whistleblowing becomes likely in organizations that actively support whistleblowing, in word and deed. These are the places with the ethics codes that lift off the page. They are likely to be high performing, relatively non-bureaucratic places, and cluster in the public rather than the private sector (Near and Miceli 1996). Norwegian public sector employees generally have a positive experience of whistleblowing, and many do so (Skivenes and Trygstad 2010). This isn't surprising. Social behaviour does not occur in a vacuum.

WEIGHING UP THE PROS AND CONS OF WHISTLEBLOWING

To become a whistleblower in health and social care services, whatever the duties of the person's professional code, requires a bit of thought. The whistleblower is raising concerns about something the organization is doing or not doing. The organization has its particular history, culture, climate and ways of managing dissent, which the whistleblower may well be very aware of. Weighing up whether or not to whistleblow becomes a sort of cost-benefit analysis (Miceli and Near 1985).

Whistleblowing involves other people, both in the organization and outside it (in health and social care, these include regulators, policy makers and politicians). The costs of not whistleblowing may well involve the perpetuation of harm, corruption and wrongdoing; the damage being done to people who are vulnerable, by virtue of their dependency on those health and social care services. The whistleblower's own personal and professional circumstances – their livelihood, career history and aspirations, their obligations and responsibilities to support others – also figure on the costs side. On the other side is the benefit that exposing harm, poor practices and wrongdoing may bring to those directly affected by it. The organization may benefit from understanding better where, tacitly or knowingly, it colluded in the harm perpetrated. The deep learning on offer to the health or social care organization, which can come from disasters in health and social care, is a benefit beyond measure. But the organization has to engage, systemically and systematically, in that process of deep learning for that benefit to be realized.

CODES AND WOES

In the UK, registered health and social care professionals hold professional obligations not to permit people using their services to come to avoidable harm. These are variously expressed in professional codes of conduct and registration. Laying a mandatory duty on health and social care staff (discussed in Chapter 6) to report poor care typically decontextualizes incidents of poor care from the situational dynamics in which they occur. Registered nurses in the UK, for example, are required by their regulatory body to raise any concerns they might have about healthcare delivery. This requirement would seem to render redundant any consideration of the pros and cons of whistleblowing – they would have to do it, wouldn't they? It seems not. Attree's interviews with 142 nurses in England (age range 21–60; length of service two weeks to 40 years; ten males) highlighted the problems they felt they faced in doing something that wasn't quite as simple as 'just report it'. What put many of these nurses off reporting, contrary to the duty of their registration to raise concerns, were fears of personal repercussions and retribution, worries about being labelled a troublemaker or being blamed for causing difficulties for colleagues. Whistleblowing was regarded as a high-risk activity with little or no pay-off for the nurse (Attree 2007).

Of course, nurses in Attree's interviews might have witnessed how those raising concerns before them had been treated. In England, the public inquiry into the failings of the Mid Staffordshire NHS Foundation Trust described the experiences of Nurse Donnelly who, in a protected disclosure under the UK's whistleblowing legislation, said she had been asked to fabricate patient nursing notes to conceal the number of patients whose length of stay in the Accident and Emergency department of Stafford Hospital was breaching the four-hour waiting time target. That is, she had been asked to lie, to make it look as though some patient waits had not been in excess of four hours. Before she disclosed, she had sought advice from her Royal College of Nursing representative, who told her that there was little that could be done, and that she should just 'keep her head down' (Francis 2013a, p.109). In other words, do nothing.

Nurse Donnelly stood out from her peers in her decision to speak up about wrongdoing. She went against the grain of the organizational culture she worked in. In general, weighing up whether to report wrongdoing hinges, in part, on the whistleblower's perceptions of the support or back-up they'll get from their immediate manager if they do. Whistleblowing is more likely in organizations that support it, and which are themselves *perceived to be* fairer and ethical (Miceli and Near 2005). An employee may be more likely to report if they think their manager will back them up. By the same token, how the employee regards organizational whistleblowing policies influences their decision to whistleblow (Sims and Keenan 1998). Supervisor support for whistleblowing, and informal policies to support external whistleblowing, are significant predictors of whistleblowing. All of these are factors directly influenced by managers in the particular organizational culture and milieu: '…organization leaders create an environment of support and encouragement for their employees to speak up and blow the whistle on illegal, unethical, or illegitimate activities' (Sims and Keenan 1998, p.420).

Key constituents of this 'environment of support and encouragement' to speak out are legal rights and protection, trade union support and communicative cultures in organizations where employees can freely voice opinion and criticism, and report wrongdoing, poor practice or corruption. In extensive studies on whistleblowing among public officials in Norway, Skivenes and Trygstad (2010) found that employees witnessing serious wrongdoing at work generally voiced their concerns and reported misconduct they observed to someone. Two-thirds of the 834 whistleblowers in this study said changes had come about as a result of their speaking out; eight out of ten reported they had had a positive response to their concerns. Employees were more likely to report misconduct if the person responsible was a subordinate or colleague, rather than an immediate supervisor or senior manager. Being a member of a trade union increased the likelihood of whistleblowing; and good contact with employee representatives increased the probability of external whistleblowing if the initial concern had not been responded to. Employees who came into frequent contact with their immediate supervisor were more likely to get a positive response to their concerns, and to be less likely to go outside the organization with their concerns (Skivenes and Trygstad 2010).

So the wider context counts when it comes to the likelihood that an employee will raise concerns. If wrongdoing is sufficiently bad, if it is observed, and if the employee thinks that by raising a concern they can stop it, *without suffering personal detriment and harm*, they are more likely to act. Employment protection, the right and support to raise concerns, and a workplace culture where it is expected, rather than mandated, that employees will raise concerns and be supported when they do, significantly influence the likelihood of reporting. Employees in Skivenes and Trygstad's study were working in the Norwegian public sector, where there is a high rate of trade union membership (86 per cent of public sector employees are unionized). In Norway, employees have a constitutional right to raise any concern not deemed confidential in law, and they have the right to report misconduct. Compared to the US and UK, these employees have strong protection against unfair dismissal. Employee rights in Norway support whistleblowing activity: 'Norwegian employees, to a great extent, perceive their whistleblowing activity as positive and effective' (Skivenes and Trygstad 2010, p.1091).

The Australian survey (Brown 2008), referred to earlier, found the decisions of public sector employees to blow the whistle were strongly influenced by the culture of their organization, as well as by the perceived seriousness of the wrongdoing and by their belief as to whether reporting the wrongdoing would serve any good purpose. Reporting was more likely when employees believed the wrongdoing was serious and frequent, when they had direct evidence of the wrongdoing, and when it affected them personally. If the wrongdoing involved a lot of people, or the perpetrators were senior to the whistleblower, then the employee was less likely to report (Brown 2008).

Reporting wrongdoing, and getting it put right, are very hard where bad or illegal practice is commonplace and tacitly tolerated, or where whistleblowing procedures feel like an obstacle course designed to trip up those bold enough to try and use them. When they are confident their concerns will be listened to, employees are more likely to speak out (Brown 2008). The main reasons for not reporting is a belief that nothing will be done about the wrongdoing, or that the employee will suffer reprisal – in other words, that the messenger will be shot while the message goes unheeded. Speaking truth to power is always a tough call.

UK WHISTLEBLOWING IN LAW

Providing legal protection to the whistleblower making a public interest disclosure has been the stated aim of statute internationally for some time. In the UK, the Public Interest Disclosure Act 1998 (PIDA) was intended to protect individuals who make certain disclosures in the public interest. Here, from a legal point of view, whistleblowing is justified if a worker has a reasonable belief that a type of wrongdoing specified in the legislation affects the public interest. In changes implemented under the Enterprise and Regulatory Reform Act 2013, UK whistleblowers have protection from victimization by co-workers, as well as employers.

In the UK, the operative provisions of PIDA are contained in Part IVA of the Employment Rights Act 1996. They apply to both the public and private sector and cover most, but not all, workers. (In 2016, members of the armed forces, intelligence services and volunteers do not have protection under the Act's provisions. Some self-employed contractors may have protection under PIDA, although most do not.) There is no statutory right to disclose in the UK, although a contractual right may exist. Types of disclosure that can give rise to employee protection are called 'qualifying disclosures' and cover matters such as where the worker reasonably believes the concern might be a crime; or where there has been a failure to comply with a legal obligation; or one concerning potential damage to the environment; or danger to the health and safety of a person. Most protection under this law is given to those who disclose information internally. However, workers can disclose to a person prescribed in the relevant regulations if they reasonably believe that the matter falls within that person's remit, and that the information and any allegation contained in it are substantially true. Wider disclosures can be made if the worker fulfils additional requirements – for example, they are not disclosing for personal gain; they have already disclosed the information to the employer (unless they believe they would suffer detriment, or the employer would destroy evidence if they were alerted). Detailed provision is also made for the external disclosure of information about exceptionally serious wrongdoing. The worker has a right not to suffer detriment for making a protected disclosure. But retaliation against the whistleblower is not a criminal offence in the UK, and it is the case that whistleblowers may find themselves vulnerable to victimization and dismissal following their speaking out.

How far these legal provisions have protected UK employees is a moot point. De Maria (2006, p.647) called whistleblowing legislation the 'state management of dissent', and it is certainly the case that a number of NHS whistleblowers have found their concerns managed by their employer without any protection from whistleblowing legislation. Lewis (2008) regarded PIDA's protection of whistleblowers as inadequate. He argued that employers should be under a statutory duty to establish and maintain effective reporting procedures; and that employers should not impose a contractual duty upon employees to report in the absence of a proper procedure. Lewis called for legislation to relieve people of civil or criminal liability if they make a protected disclosure. Disclosures are only protected if the person reasonably believes them to be correct: should that reasonable belief turn out to be incorrect, defamation proceedings can be brought against a worker making the disclosure. That person might then have to rely on the defence of qualified privilege (which permits certain persons to make statements that would be considered slander or libel if made by anyone else). Lewis (2008) has suggested that a defence of absolute privilege should be available to the whistleblower, as well as specific statutory protection against post-employment detriment

– for example, an employer refusing to provide a reference for the whistleblower.

As it stands, PIDA is convoluted law. A person contemplating making a protected disclosure under it is well-advised to take legal advice before, and not after, raising the concern. The Health Committee of the House of Commons acknowledged some of the Act's limitations. While PIDA is supposed to provide protection against employee detriment, and its effect to be deterrent rather than restorative, its complexity is such that success in a case brought under PIDA can by no means be guaranteed (Pattenden 2003; HOC 2015).

Over and above the provisions and limits of this particular statute, there are contrasting opinions on what whistleblowing legislation and duties exist for. One perspective is that of the employee acting in line with their individual conscience to counter wrongdoing (like, say, the heroic slayer of a mythical dragon). Less seductive, is the view that whistleblowing statute serves as a management tool to control the workforce (Tsahuridu and Vandekerckhove 2008). The first view regards whistleblower protection as promoting individual responsibility and autonomy in the workplace. The second understands whistleblower protection to be *de facto* protective cover for the organization, as it offloads responsibility for holding the moral compass in the workplace from employer onto employee.

In evidence to the Health Committee of the UK House of Commons (HOC 2015), the chief executive of the UK charity PCaW said that PIDA acted more as a deterrent than a remedy: if an employee has to have recourse to PIDA's provisions, then his or her employment prospects are already substantially impaired. Organizational whistleblowing policies may use PIDA as a legal firewall – do this, at the right time, in the right way, in the right sequence, or face the consequences, if you fancy your chances taking us on.

PARADOXES IN WHISTLEBLOWING POLICY AND PROCEDURES

To be used and useful, people need to know about, understand and have confidence in an organization's whistleblowing policy, and in those who manage it. It requires a lot of the employee, in fulfilling their side of the employment contract, when they find they have to negotiate, with all the care of someone ploughing a field of activated landmines, the tripwires of their employer's whistleblowing policy and procedures. When organizations have a whistleblowing policy in place solely to meet compliance, regulatory or legal requirements – as a procedural fig leaf we might say – the tacit suppression, discouragement or punishment of dissent is experienced as the organizational *actualité*, whatever the policy says.

Vandekerckhove (2011) identified five paradoxes in managing whistleblowing. The first is the truism that all the grand talk about whistleblowing protection doesn't always get – that whistleblowing policies work best in organizations that don't really need them; that is to say, in places where early corrective action is taken, where and when needed. Kaptein (2008) put forward seven features of an ethical organizational culture, which were:

1. clarity (of normative expectations laid on employees)

2. congruency (with these expectations) by managers

3. feasibility (how far the organization creates the conditions that enable employees to meet the expectations)

4. supportability (how far the organization creates support mechanisms to meet expectations)

5. transparency (employees can only be held accountable if they knew the consequences of their actions)

6. discussability (the opportunity employees have to raise concerns and issues)

7. sanctionability (enforcement of sanctions to wrongdoing, rather than turning a blind eye).

Organizations delivering on these ethical dimensions are not going to need to rely on the paraphernalia of policy, procedures, helplines for whistleblowers and all the rest – but they will have all of that because they manifest ethical virtues that deal with problems before they threaten the organization, and the people it serves.

Vandekerckhove's second paradox concerns anonymous reporting channels – something that whistleblowers often say they want but which don't always help. Hunton and Rose (2011), for instance, found that anonymous reports were seen as less credible by managers receiving them, and fewer resources were allocated to investigating and rectifying reported wrongdoing.

The third paradox lies in rectifying the problem the whistleblower raises, which may itself create other problems for the organization's managers. The stakes are higher if the whistleblowing matter threatens the organization; if it does, whistleblowing is less likely to be effective (Near and Miceli 1995). The fourth paradox is the loose procedural talk about the *right* to blow the whistle, whereas it is, in reality, an implied or disguised duty, as the House of Commons committee referred to earlier made clear. When an issue blows up, those who knew but did not report it are judged, blamed and held to account, no matter what fear of reprisal they may have had about raising the concern in the first place. The right becomes a liability. The fifth paradox is the response to whistleblowing and to the employee raising concerns: this itself can lead to detriment, reprisal and wrongdoing *against the employee*. These paradoxes are in perfect symmetry: the employee is damned if they do, and damned if they don't.

WHAT HAPPENS WHEN PEOPLE WHISTLEBLOW?

The outlook isn't always a rosy one for the whistleblower. There is no certainty that anything will change after a whistleblower has put themselves through the procedural mill to raise their concerns. Momentary acclaim for being the heroic martyr who took on the iron cage of a dehumanized bureaucracy won't pay bills, repair relationships or develop new careers if the whistleblower finds themselves dealing with career ruin, bankruptcy, depression or alcoholism (Alford 2001; Rothschild and Miethe 1999).

The UK House of Commons Committee of Public Accounts, having taken evidence from four government departments (Education; Health; Revenue and Customs, Ministry of Defence), observed in its 2014 report on whistleblowing that '…whistleblowers who have come forward have had to show remarkable bravery' (HOC 2014, p.3). It commented that the treatment of some whistleblowers had been 'shocking', with whistleblowers sometimes left unprotected from victimization. The Committee noted the 'startling disconnect between the generally good quality of whistleblowing policies in theory and how arrangements actually work in practice' (HOC 2014, p.6).

When taking evidence for this report on whistleblowing, the chair of the UK House of Commons Public Accounts Committee (PAC) remarked:

> I will just say that we tried to get a number of whistleblowers whose evidence has been proven credible to come and talk to us about their experience… We had somebody from HMRC [Her Majesty's Revenue and Customs] who would not come, somebody from the MOD [Ministry of Defence] who would not come, somebody from local government who would not come, and also somebody from the police. That shows there is still a culture of complete fear out there…which demonstrates the difficulties that we are facing. (PAC 2014)

Giving evidence before the PAC, Kay Sheldon, who had been a board member of the Care Quality Commission (CQC), the health and care regulator in England, described some her experiences of whistleblowing to the CQC:

> …I started to raise some quite serious concerns about CQC – about the leadership, the management and the culture. I felt that the organisation was at risk of not fulfilling its statutory duties, so they were really quite serious concerns. Unfortunately, because the culture was quite oppressive, those concerns were not well received. The more I tried to get them taken seriously, the more I was subject to inappropriate behaviour, such as being excluded from roles that had been agreed. My mental health was questioned. I am obviously open about the fact that I have had mental health issues, but that was used against me. A secret mental health report was done on me…

As I was really very concerned that the organisation was failing, and failing patients – people who use services – I felt that I had to go outside the organisation. I approached the National Audit Office, the Department of Health and the Mid Staffs public inquiry, and it was the inquiry that responded positively... [U]nbeknown to me, the chair of the Care Quality Commission wrote to (Secretary of State for Health) asking for me to be removed. I did not know that had happened. I was called into the Department of Health and told that there was going to be an independent review, and I was asked not to attend any further board meetings. It was pretty clear to me that they wanted me out of the picture as fast as possible, so I declined. I said I wanted to continue going to board meetings, which I did. I had someone with me, because I knew that would be necessary.

The review that was set up was not independent; I think that is the thing to say. Frankly, it was a deliberate hatchet job; there is no other way to describe it. I met with the person doing the review for about an hour, and I was told it was going to report within 10 days, but it didn't. It dragged on. I didn't hear anything else, but when I got my personal data, I found out that the person doing the review, the CQC and the Department of Health were in quite a lot of contact. I was completely out of it. I didn't have a voice. (PAC 2014)

Asked if she thought her concerns would be dealt with differently (than they were in 2011–2012), Kay Sheldon was unconvinced they would be:

I am not convinced, because of the extreme things that happened – the fact that I did raise some very serious issues and really all they were intent on was to get rid of me. I don't think the Department of Health and the officials there have really taken responsibility for what happened. Personally, I think that if they did – if they did engage with me or other whistleblowers – that would really help to change things, but so far they haven't done it, frankly. (PAC 2014)

As the messenger taking the hit for her message, Kay Sheldon was subjected to referral, without her knowledge, for psychiatric assessment. Sheldon recounted her short conversation with the director of a private occupational health service paid by the Department of Health to carry out this covert, Kafkaesque assessment:

> ...(the Chair of the CQC) told me that I had been referred to this occupational health company, Medigold, which I was quite surprised about. I phoned up simply to cancel the appointment and had a 10-minute conversation to say, 'I don't think I need to see a doctor, but a bit of support would be nice.'

> After that 10-minute conversation with the owner of Medigold, he wrote this three-page letter saying that I probably had paranoid schizophrenia and that he would speak in confidence to the medical director and that my medical notes should be obtained in confidence. I just discovered this in my personal data. I did not know. (PAC 2014)

Sheldon's account of her experiences at the hands of a government regulator highlights a number of typical retaliations that may be visited on the whistleblower after they raise their concerns. First is an allegation or vague innuendo that questions the whistleblower's mental health status ('mental health problems run in the family'... 'she was always difficult'...). Second are the shadowy, behind-the-scenes, not quite in daylight, machinations of the organization or government department, aimed at reconstructing the reality the whistleblower speaks out about, thus closing down the disclosures and marginalizing the person making them, before they have been heard. Third are the systemic 'blind eye' or 'deaf ear' responses (discussed in the following chapter) of other responsible organizations, who turn away from the disclosures, or turn upon the person making them.

RETALIATION AND RETRIBUTION

A whistleblower is well advised to entertain the possibility – indeed the expectation – that their organization, whatever its public proclamations and statutory obligations to whistleblowers, will react harshly to them, the messenger, before turning attention to the message they bring. The nature and extent of retaliation has nothing to do with any personal characteristics of the whistleblower (Near and Miceli 1996), even though *ad hominem* attacks on their character, honesty and competence are not uncommon.

The more serious the allegation the whistleblower makes, the more likely it is that they will suffer detriment. Kay Sheldon's experience at the hands of the CQC and Department of Health, recounted above, is testimony to this. The whistleblower is at greater risk of detriment when the wrongdoing they allege is very serious; when the investigation was inconclusive; and when more than one person was implicated in the wrongdoing. Retaliation is more likely if the matter goes outside the organization (external whistleblowing), or when those accused of wrongdoing work at a higher organizational grade than the whistleblower. In these circumstances, vengeance is more likely to be exacted on the whistleblower (Brown 2008).

Retaliation has been described as 'taking an undesirable action against a whistleblower – in direct response to the whistleblowing – who reported wrongdoing internally or externally, outside the organization' (Rehg *et al.* 2008, p.222). Retaliation can be informal, official, overt or covert. Even though legal protection for the whistleblower exists across many jurisdictions internationally, Tsahuridu (2011) observed that retaliation, threats and retribution seem to have increased, even as whistleblowing protection has grown. Retaliatory acts are not minor slights or insignificant trifles. The litany of loss that may be the lot of the whistleblower includes losing their job (being sacked, forced to resign or retire early); being blacklisted; getting a poor performance evaluation *after* they blew the whistle; increased management surveillance of their work; being criticized or given the cold shoulder by colleagues. The risk profile that the whistleblower establishes is not one that many organizations want to absorb (Rothschild and Miethe 1999). A whistleblower spells trouble.

The severity of the backlash is greater if the whistleblower is not a supervisor or manager, if they go outside the organization to raise their concern, or if they blow the whistle on something serious (Hedin and Månsson 2012; Jos, Tompkins and Hays 1989; Rothschild and Miethe 1999). Referral to a psychiatrist is not uncommon (as in the case of Kay Sheldon discussed above), resulting in the whistleblower being diagnosed with a mental illness (the murky label of 'personality disorder' proves popular) that will inevitably scupper any future chance the employee has of resuming, still less progressing in, their profession, sector or job of choice. Official reprisals such as demotion, and legal or quasi-legal retribution such as surveillance, the scouring of historic expense claims for minute discrepancies that were previously passed for payment, are the familiar *modi operandi* of an organization in witch hunter mode, a far cry from the 'lessons have been learned', 'changes have been made' pronouncements of those in charge of the organization *after* a disaster has come to public attention (Ash 2011, 2013).

Organizational management of dissent has many means of silencing in its toolkit. Official channels, such as the use of organizational grievance procedures or the courts, may offer the promise of justice to the employee, but achieving justice is compromised when the vast power resources of the organization are mobilized against the whistleblower, who may find they are in danger of losing their home as a consequence of their whistleblowing. Dissent can effectively be neutralized by, for example, setting up inquiries, reviews and investigations that are prolonged and protracted, exhausting public patience and attention. Tony Blair, past UK Prime Minister and himself no stranger to controversy, offered private (subsequently published) advice on disaster management to Rebekah Brooks, then chief executive of the global media conglomerate News Corporation. At the time, Brooks was under intense public scrutiny for her role in phone-hacking by the Murdoch-owned tabloid press in the UK. In an email to her boss James Murdoch on 11 July 2011, Brooks said Blair gave her this advice to manage the maelstrom she found herself in:

> 1. Form an independent unit that has a outside junior counsel…a great and good type, a serious forensic criminal barrister, internal counsel, proper fact checkers, etc. in it. Get them to investigate (Brooks) and others and publish a…report. 2. Publish part one of the report at same time as the police closes its inquiry and clear you and accept shortcomings and new solutions and process and part two when any trials are over. (Rebekah Brooks, email on Tony Blair's advice, *The Guardian* 2014)

From the point of view of the corporation, Blair's (presumably *pro bono*) advice to Brooks was a masterclass in dissent management and blowing out the critical voices. In the event, Brooks and her employers marshalled many million pounds' worth of top-end legal counsel; Brooks was acquitted of five charges of phone-hacking, conspiracy to commit misconduct in a public office, and to pervert the course of justice, relating to her time as editor of two UK tabloids and as head of the Murdoch-owned company (Davies 2014). People making allegations prior to this case, including many in the public eye, had been subjected to sustained intrusion and vitriol in critical media coverage of their lives, sustained over many years. This is, of course, the type of retaliation that some people raising concerns about the NHS have suffered and where, again, millions of pounds (of public money) have been spent on legal fees to manage dissent, by silencing it (Campbell 2014).

FACING INTO FEAR

Using fear as a weapon to silence is very effective. In the public inquiry into the failings of the Mid Staffordshire NHS Foundation Trust in England, one of the people to speak out at Stafford Hospital was Nurse Donnelly, who was referred to above. Described as 'a most impressive and courageous witness' by Robert Francis, the chair of the public inquiry, Nurse Donnelly had at first been reluctant to complain about fabricated patient records, for fear of repercussions (Francis 2013a, p.235). Her fears were well-founded. In her evidence to the inquiry, Nurse Donnelly described being harassed by colleagues, being threatened, and:

> …people were saying, 'Oh, you shouldn't have done this, you shouldn't have spoken out.' And then physical threats were made in terms of people saying that I needed to – again, watch myself while I was walking to my car at the end of a shift. People saying that they know where I live, and basically threats to, sort of, my physical safety were made, to the point where…at the end of a shift…at night I would have to have either my mum or my dad or my husband come and collect me from work because I was too afraid to walk to my car in the dark on my own.

Nurse Donnelly described how this threatening behaviour continued after she had reported her concerns:

> It was slightly more subversive and I think people were slightly more guarded in how they were doing it. You know, on one particular occasion another staff nurse followed me into the toilet which was also our locker room and locked the door behind her, locking me in, and demanded to know if I had a problem with her and if I was going to say anything about her, and basically threatening me not to do so if I did… So people were still doing things, but not so publicly… They were doing it slightly more discreetly… (Francis 2013a, p.236)

Nurse Donnelly resigned from her job in Mid Staffordshire NHS Foundation Trust some time after she had faced out her fears of retaliation. Staying in or returning to their job is not something that many NHS whistleblowers get to do, whatever their wish. Dr Phil Hammond, an England-based registered medical doctor and journalist, has supported many NHS whistleblowers since 1992. None has returned to their job or previous employment (Hammond 2015). It took Dr Stephen Bolsin, the consultant anaesthetist at the Bristol Royal Infirmary (BRI) who raised concerns about death rates of children undergoing heart surgery, six years to get his concerns heard and to see a drop in mortality rates. Bolsin became the butt of considerable hostility from consultant paediatric surgeons at the BRI; his concerns were ignored until he took these to the media.

THE SMELL OF SALEM

When retaliation is significant, the whistleblower pays what (Alford 2001, p.10) said were '…the terrible costs of going up against the organization, costs most of us are not even aware of because they are not apparent until one crosses an invisible line'. The whistleblower may find themselves subjected to small, individually minor, but collectively destructive acts of victimization in the aftermath of their raising concerns. These can become witch hunts with the smell of Salem about them.

The US Government Accountability Project (GAP), an American non-profit, non-partisan, public interest law firm that has provided legal representation to many US whistleblowers, including Edward Snowden, commented that, 'The uglier the tactic, the more effective it is at silencing critics and scaring off anyone else who might challenge abuses of power' (Devine and Devine 2010, p.7). Pernicious silencing tactics include bringing conflict of interests charges against the whistleblower – for example:

- alleging the whistleblower was doing the very same act that they are complaining about

- raiding the whistleblower's home to seize computers and electronic devices

- telling the whistleblower they must remain silent

- attempting prosecution for alleged false statements solely based on hearsay allegation by a mediator sworn to confidentiality

- unsupported allegations of mental illness, revenge, depression, drug misuse

- prolonged garden leave

- blacklisting and whispering campaigns of many years' duration

- classifying information years after the fact and then charging the whistleblower *post hoc* with disclosure of sensitive information

- the 'smokescreen syndrome' (kicking up sand about an unrelated and irrelevant matter to take attention away from the disclosure).

This GAP report concluded that, 'Exoneration does not free whistleblowers from retaliation unless they get the point and become silent observers after successfully defending their innocence' (Devine and Devine 2010, p.9). Put up, shut up, or face the consequences.

OSTRACISM AND OUTCASTS

It can get worse, but forewarned is forearmed for the whistleblower. 'Death', 'denial' and 'destruction' are epithets that pepper research reports and personal accounts of whistleblowing and its impacts. Perry described the act of whistleblowing as 'occupational suicide', causing 'accidental career death' on the downward spiral that can be the post-disclosure trajectory (Perry 1998, pp.235, 240, 241). Williams (2001, p.19) likened the ostracism of whistleblowers to a 'social death'. Alford (2001, p.38) heard whistleblowers he spoke with describe 'living in the position of the dead'.

If not physical death, there is a sobering list of what a whistleblower needs to be prepared for when they raise concerns. These include, in no particular order of unpleasantness: social ostracism, harassment, muck-raking and rumour-spreading; threats; reprimands; referral to psychiatrists; blocking of appointments and promotions; forced job transfers; being given impossible tasks to do and then failing; denial of work opportunities to progress, even to function; formal reprimands for minor matters; legal action; dismissal; blacklisting; physical assault (Martin 2013). Leaning in to face out that lot is a big task.

A very common reprisal against whistleblowers is social ostracism, a hugely powerful, deeply destructive psychological phenomenon with irreparable, often lifelong, consequences for the individual. Co-workers, individually or collectively, shun the whistleblower, closing down the informal, everyday social pleasantries of work life, socially isolating them and erecting a wall of critical or contemptuous silence. Petty harassment, taking the whistleblower's belongings, sabotaging their work space, removing access to facilities, are at the milder end of a spectrum that may include spreading malicious rumour, spite, vicious personal attacks, casting innuendo, discrediting and bad-mouthing the whistleblower, circulating damaging information, and general denunciation. Counter-charges may be brought, fabricated to inflict maximum damage and suffering on the whistleblower – for example, accusations of sexual harassment and, of course, mental disorder. It may take months or years before these are considered, and then dropped because of lack of evidence (Hedin and Månsson 2012; Martin 2013; Williams 2001).

Being ostracized and ignored violates some fundamental human needs. The human sense and need for personal connection to others is severed, as is the connection between one's actions and their outcomes. Personal self-esteem is traduced, and becomes infected with shame, confusion and self-doubt. Existentially, the person ostracized ceases to feel they exist. They experience being invisible, mute and unheard. Violation of such deep human needs has consequences for a person's psychological survival beyond the aftermath of the whistleblowing. And these consequences extend far wider than the individual. They affect the ostracizers, the workplace team or group, and the way the organization works together:

> ...when a whistleblower is ostracized, the effect is detrimental to the entire organization because of low morale, low productivity, job turnover, and rehiring and retraining costs. The effects of ostracism may be harmful at a societal level as well. (Williams 2001, p.205)

Ostracism is a powerful and pernicious propensity of workplace and social life. People want to belong, to fit in and be part of the group. Achieving this comes at a price as, 'in order to belong, and be included, we conform, comply, obey, engage in groupthink, stereotype out-groups, and inhibit prosocial tendencies' (Williams 2001, p.258). When these behavioural and psychological forces are marshalled against the whistleblower, their sense of belonging, self-control, self-esteem and meaningful existence is quickly stripped away. Added to which, the whistleblower may struggle with the double bind that is their professional code of practice requiring them to disclose corrupt or bad practice. This malpractice may be rooted in (if not caused by) complex contextual problems in health and social care organizations – for example, the tacit political sanctioning of inferior care by constant, prolonged under-resourcing of services (Hedin and Månsson 2012). In the double bind that is speaking out, the employee carries the can, whether they raise a concern or not. And, as the following chapter explores, it is the organizational culture in which they work that profoundly influences what happens to the whistleblower when they speak out.

CHAPTER 3

ORGANIZATIONAL CULTURE AND THE WHISTLEBLOWER

Understanding why it is that whistleblowers may be ignored, disbelieved or scapegoated when they raise concerns, calls for a dig deep into the dynamics of health and social care systems and organizations, and into the individual and social interactions and relationships that exist within them. This chapter looks at aspects of organizational culture, and its superordinate power to mould and shape the behaviour and actions of people working in health and social care services. This is the culture to which, and within which, the whistleblower discloses. Organizational culture can constrain or support, punish or reward, employees speaking out about corrupt, bad or unlawful practice. Whatever its public statements, an organization that sends out no *meaningful* signals about its commitment to ethical practice and its expectation that every employee (and not just those holding a professional registration) must work to deliver ethical care, is not an ethical organization.

To consider organizational culture and cultures, and the actions of a whistleblower within these, this chapter first considers what organizational 'climate' and 'culture' mean, and how various 'layers' of culture coexist, and not always harmoniously, within health and social care systems. 'Undiscussable' aspects of organizational life, and the whistleblower's action in bringing these into the open, are discussed. The second section looks at how wrongdoing becomes normalized, and at how socialization into ways of working in a team or department can mean that poor or harmful practice becomes rationalized, and the metaphorical blind eye or deaf ear is turned away from the wrongdoing. This discussion expands to consider the ethics of human agency, or moral agency, where a person with the ability to speak out or stay silent in the face of wrongdoing uses a standard of 'right' or 'wrong'. The final section looks at the actions and behaviour of groups in the workplace. It discusses the capacity of a minority to influence group thinking, alongside the power of the group to close down, or put off limits, wider examination of the consequences of decisions it reaches. As a whole, the chapter aims to open the space within which we can see the actions of the whistleblower, and to take in examination of social relations, organizational cultures and their influence on ethical practice in the workplace. Inevitably, it is hard to escape the mixing of metaphors in this discussion, be they bad apples, elephants in the room, the emperor's clothes, eyes that do not see or ears that do not hear. Sometimes the language of myth, metaphor and gallows humour signals where it is we need to lean in and look harder at what goes on in organizations, and at the part the whistleblower plays in bringing some of that to light.

ORGANIZATIONAL CLIMATE AND CULTURE

What people do, and how they experience their job and their workplace, whatever their pay grade, is influenced by the climate and the culture of the organization. 'Organizational climate' and 'organizational culture' – distinct yet overlapping concepts for understanding how people experience their workplace – describe aspects of work that are the invisible bedfellows of all the 'how-to' apparatus of the organization's operations, such as its standards, targets and rituals of performance management. Schneider and Barbera (2014) have gone so far as to claim that everything happening in an organization influences, and is influenced by, organizational climate and culture, implying that the external inputs into an organization – resources, policy, intellectual capital and the rest – are secondary to the way employees work to process those inputs, and the way the organization is perceived and experienced by them.

Organizational 'climate' can be described as those 'shared and enduring perceptions of psychologically important aspects of a particular work environment' (Morrison and Milliken 2000, p.714), or the behaviours that are expected, supported and rewarded, and the shared meanings employees attach to them.

Organizational 'culture', on the other hand, is:

> ...a pattern of shared basic assumptions learned by a group as it solved problems of external adaptation and internal integration, which has worked well enough to be considered valid and, therefore, to be taught to new members as the correct way to perceive, think, and feel in relation to those problems. (Schein 2010, p.18)

The 'teaching' that Schein talks about here is not the courses, workshops or induction programmes employees may embark upon. Rather it is the implicit, intangible, affective ways in which people in the organization talk to each other, about each other and about the organization, and the messages and stories that convey this to a new recruit. Socialization into shared meanings and basic assumptions about the work and the workplace are conveyed in the directions, decisions and actions of leaders and managers, and the stories and tales of organizational life that are transmitted in the rite of passage that is workplace orientation. Culture – present in each dynamic moment of organizational life – is the background operating system of work. It shapes, constrains and defines behaviour and interactions with others. Its importance to whistleblowing, to speaking out, or to walking on by, cannot be underestimated. The whistleblower is often the one who acts counter-culturally to say 'the emperor is without clothes'. For that, they may pay a price.

LAYERS OF CULTURE

Any organization operates within a bigger frame – be that global, national, political, economic, legal. Within health and social care systems, such as the NHS and social care services, there are subcultures (among different professional or occupational groups, or different organizational functions, such as finance or audit), and micro-cultures (for example, within local teams or workgroups). For Schein (2010), there were three layers of organizational culture. First are the 'artefacts', or those structures and processes that are observable. You can see, feel, hear them. They include human interactions, group norms, ways of doing things, habits of thinking, shared meanings, stories, what gets celebrated, remarked upon, remembered. Second are espoused values and goals, as well as rationalizations such as 'turning the blind eye' to bad practice, or the shortcuts and workarounds adopted get the job done. These may or may not be congruent with the artefacts. Third are underlying assumptions, those unconscious, taken-for-granted beliefs and values that influence thoughts, feelings and perception. These underlying assumptions don't often get expression in the day-to-day life of organizations. They may be what everyone 'knows', but no one talks about, or does anything about. These assumptions are mostly undiscussable. That is, everyone knows, but no one says, until the whistleblower speaks out.

UNDISCUSSABLES OF ORGANIZATIONAL LIFE

These 'undiscussables' – major obstacles to organizational learning – are covert processes usually hidden from everyday awareness (Marshak 2006). Many of the 'undiscussables' (Argyris 1980, 1986, 1990) are topics that are avoided by the organization and groups working in it. Their avoidance, and those avoided topics, are not discussed. Such hidden dimensions and unconscious dynamics of organizational change are processes *known* about and apparent in tacit, shared assumptions. Cultural expectations and norms of etiquette, tact and politeness mean that the undiscussables remain undiscussed. They are the elephant in the room, of which none can speak. Instead, people step carefully around it, rearrange the furniture and open the window.

Organizational cultures exert a powerful hold on keeping these undiscussables undiscussable. Predominant mindsets in the organization – the 'theories in use' or the thinking models that prevail (Schein 2010) – may arise as defensive *modi operandi* that shape reaction and response. These may reward *anti*-learning, that is, behaviours that are superficial, defensive, fire-fighting, blaming and denying. Argyris called these 'self-sealing processes' (Noonan 2007); their effect is to corrode trust and transparency in the organization. Self-sealing processes close off and then close down deep thinking and reflection about work. They discourage detachment from the minute 'stuff' of human interaction (witnessed in the who-did-what-to-whom, he-said, she-said chatter-noise of social engagement), and seal off the possibility of larger-scale reflection on change. The mindless repetition by organizational leaders that 'lessons will be learned' and 'we take these matters very seriously' when serious harm comes to light publicly, is a self-sealing reaction. It closes down reflective, detached and deep thinking and analysis of what goes wrong, what could go wrong, and why that is.

Egan called these covert processes the shadow side of an organization. Rather like a seldom-glimpsed underbelly of the elephant in the room, the shadow side is:

> ...all the important activities and arrangements that do not get identified, discussed, and managed in decision-making forums that can make a difference. The shadow side deals with the covert, the undiscussed, the undiscussable, and the unmentionable. It includes arrangements not found in organizational manuals and company documents or on organizational charts. (Egan 1994, p.4)

These covert processes operate alongside the explicit, overt, public and official face, or façade, of the organization. The shadow side is a feature of human interaction, of people working together. It isn't the performance targets, the annual report, all the policies and procedures people in the organization have to sign up to and comply with at work. That overt, or top-note, paraphernalia exists in covert duality with the shadow side. Strategy, directives, policies, budgets, job titles and organization charts are 'out there'; trust, jealously, rivalry, sabotage, spite, power struggles, ambition, fear, insecurity, the grapevine and gossip are invisible processes 'in here'. Targets, plans and what is in the public domain are the rational explicits; people, emotions, feelings, the-what-really-happens, are covert implicits. All of the shadow side is, by definition, out of focus. The whistleblower may bring it into view when they raise concerns.

The scandal that was Winterbourne View in England illustrated this. This registered, regulated place run by a private company was set up to provide assessment and treatment to around 20 adults with learning disabilities. It operated for barely five years before being closed down after a BBC TV programme broadcast footage of some adults being badly harmed by some people who worked there. Except that 'badly harmed' doesn't quite capture what looked from the outside like institutionalized cruelty, debasement and brutality towards people who were vulnerable, without anyone there to look out for them, and protect them from the sadism of some people paid to provide this so-called assessment and treatment.

Soon after this segregated, purpose-built unit opened up, reports and allegations of abuse, mistreatment and harm were passed to the local area safeguarding service, and the statutory regulator of this facility. Agencies receiving these reports took weeks to respond or investigate. When they did, whatever actions those paid to run Winterbourne View were supposed to carry out were never subject to time limits. Within weeks of starting work there in 2010 the whistleblower, Terry Bryan, raised serious concerns with the hospital and the local safeguarding board (SGASB 2012). Time passed. The cruelty continued. Terry Bryan took his concerns to the BBC (BBC 2011). The BBC *Panorama* programme, filmed undercover and broadcast in May 2011, led to this vicious mockery of care and treatment being closed down, with criminal charges brought and convictions secured against those who assaulted some of the isolated and terrorized human beings who had to live there. Winterbourne View encapsulated an institutionalized denial, through dilatoriness, of 'undiscussables' – the capacity of people with power to inflict unbearable pain and suffering, systematically and without challenge, on those less powerful than themselves.

Argyris (1990) believed that when organizational leaders learned how to address the undiscussables, they developed the capacity to have robust conversations that didn't shy away from the matter in hand, be that the elephant in the room or the whistleblower's concerns (which may be the same thing). The pressures and demands of running health and social care services can mean getting the job done, even though 'everyone knows' shortcuts are being made, day after day, and that shoestrings are ever nearer to snapping – conditions that are not so much undiscussable as normalized. People, whether leaders, managers, clinicians, professionals or staff became skilful in constructing workarounds. Even though everyday workarounds are known about, they are a way of navigating round the problem, a tacit cover-up. Argyris called this 'skilled incompetence' because it produces what is unintended and it does this repeatedly, without any direction being issued. The blind eye is turned. And turned again. Argyris said this 'fancy footwork' enabled the organization to sidestep contentious issues, but at a cost. The cost is the silencing of the employees, who stop questioning or challenging (Argyris 1990) – until the whistleblower comes along, that is.

FRAGMENTED CULTURES

Organizational culture is powerful, but it is not a unified monolith. Most organizations, and certainly one as large as the NHS, have differentiated subcultures, or fragmented cultures. Fragmentation exists when:

> [a] lack of clarity, multiple meanings and beliefs, and weak organizational leadership...produce complex and chaotic situations. Under such conditions, cultural manifestations are subject to divergent interpretations and organizational identity tends to become transitory and subject to opportunistic definition. (Aldrich and Ruef 2006, p.126)

In large organizations such as local councils and the NHS, subcultures are often associated with different professional groups or occupations – for example, in healthcare, ambulance service workers, consultants, healthcare professionals, junior doctors, nurses, radiologists, social workers, support and ancillary staff, as well as management hierarchies. In 2014 the King's Fund, an independent charity working to improve health and healthcare in England, surveyed culture and 'compassionate care' in the NHS. Over 2000 responses indicated a mixed picture of leadership and culture in NHS England. There was a consistent and significant discrepancy between the responses executive directors gave, and those of other NHS staff, particularly nurses and doctors. The vast majority of executive directors (84%) said their organization manifested openness, honesty and challenge, in contrast to just 37 per cent of doctors and 31 per cent of nurses who thought the same. Overall, fewer than four out of ten (39%) of staff believed their part of the NHS was characterized by openness, honesty and challenge. As for raising concerns, nearly all executives (94%) in this survey said they were able to raise any concerns they had about quality and care, compared to 66 per cent of doctors and 57 per cent of nurses (those delivering healthcare). The King's Fund concluded that these survey results '…consistently revealed a difference between the views of executive board members and the rest of their organisations. This suggests that boards are not in tune with how staff are feeling about their organisation' (King's Fund 2014, p.10).

The findings of the King's Fund survey were not out of synch with work done elsewhere. In a US survey of three firms (in the finance sector; manufacturing; a public utility), Treviño, Weaver and Brown (2008) found senior manager perceptions about ethical practice in the organization to be significantly more positive, compared to the more negative views of lower-level or pay-grade employees. These authors observed that 'it's lovely at the top'.

There is rather more to this, though, than senior managers wearing rose-tinted glasses, oblivious to life on the shop floor of health or social care services. In relation to whistleblowing in the NHS, a more discernable, that is pervasive, belief about the ethics of work and of the NHS culture, has emerged. People working in NHS England interviewed as part of the *Freedom to Speak Up* review carried out by Robert Francis QC (Francis 2015), spoke of the *disincentive* to speak out, and of not having the stomach to raise concerns because they had seen what had happened to others who had done that before them, or that the bullying culture itself blocked expression of concerns they had (Vandekerckhove and Rumyantseva 2014).

Another common theme in responses from NHS staff who spoke to the *Freedom to Speak Up* review was that problems often arose, or persisted, because of blocks at middle management level of their unit or department. Some whistleblower interviewees said that senior managers had been wrongly briefed by HR (human resources) or by a chief nurse about their concerns; or that a newly-appointed chief executive was just not powerful enough to challenge and change the attitude or behaviour of middle managers. An NHS Director of Workforce quoted in this survey confirmed that:

Much of the feedback that I receive from staff and their representatives is that staff who have access to the very senior levels of management, usually are fairly comfortable with voicing their concerns and their opinions at that most senior level of management. It tends to be more at the middle level of management where there is a sticking point. (Vandekerckhove and Rumyantseva 2014, p.44)

NHS whistleblowers, unlike those in other sectors such as banking and finance, are likely to be suspended from work while an investigation, sometimes lasting years, is carried out. When this happens, a clinician's career can end as they cannot maintain the CPD (continuing professional development) requirements that their professional registration requires. Whistleblowers may be bullied. As one observed, 'This isn't just about whistleblowing, this is about if you disagree with me I'm in a position of power, I'm going to treat you so badly that you leave...' (Vandekerckhove and Rumyantseva 2014, p.45). The *Freedom to Speak Up* review identified old-style command and control leadership styles and structures driving and being driven by a target-riven culture of fire-fighting and cost-control. All this easily extinguishes, if it hasn't suffocated at birth, the values-based, compassionate, people-focused leadership that could tackle the undiscussables head-on. Running a few courses on compassionate care for time-pressed, stressed, target-mangled nurses doesn't quite get the problem, nor offer any solution (Carroll 2015).

SOCIALIZATION, RATIONALIZATION, NORMALIZATION

Turning the 'blind eye', or not seeing, has the effect of normalizing wrongdoing. Its perpetrators and observers are socialized to cease to regard the practice as wrong. They no longer see it. In health and social care, services are mostly delivered by teams, in groups or in conjunction with others. Methods of socialization – the informal ways and means of incorporating employees into the what and how of organizational operations – involve communication, modelling, reinforcement and direction, and occasionally sanction. Co-optation rewards employee acceptance of unethical behaviours and practices that may become unethical; and in a process of incrementalism, commitment to wrongdoing escalates over time. Compromise, where a lesser wrongdoing is justified as acceptable as it is less bad than some other act, and coercion, both fasten the socialized practice into the way things are done (Anand, Ashforth and Joshi 2004). Fitting in and conforming with workplace norms influences whether people will raise concerns about observed wrongdoing, and if they believe anything could be done if they did (Miceli and Near 1992; Near *et al.* 2004). An understandably anonymous letterwriter to *The Guardian* newspaper, who was employed by a Housing Association in the UK, called this the FIFO (fit in or fuck off) rule of organizational life (*The Guardian* 2015).

Fitting in with the team isn't a one-way ticket. Conformity in groups – 'changes in beliefs and behaviour that a member of a group may undergo as a result of pressure from one or more of the group' – can be functional or dysfunctional (Kiesler and Kiesler 1969, p.3, cited in Schminke *et al.* 2002, p.274). When one person's views differ from those of the group, that person is more likely to move towards the majority group view. If this doesn't happen, the group is more likely to reject the deviant group member. People determine right or wrong through the expectations others hold, rather than through internal sets of values. Their responses are malleable; they shift in the situation and in response to the leadership and norms created, maintained and sustained in work groups (Schminke *et al.* 2002).

Socialization and rationalization are key processes and practices at work in the normalization of whistleblowing. Rationalization has been described as the 'process by which individuals who engage in corrupt acts use socially constructed accounts to legitimate the acts in their own eyes' (Ashforth and Anand 2003, p.3). This process, or processes, for the most part remain unexamined, and employees may come to believe the rationalizations themselves. Socialization and rationalization into negative or unethical workplace norms reinforce each other, and are very hard to reverse once they are in place: they become fixed (Anand *et al.* 2004). A social cocoon develops where, like bubble-wrap, socialization processes insulate those protected within them. This protection is made up of co-optation, incrementalism and compromise; people are co-opted into ways of working in order to get on with the job; poor practices are adopted incrementally; and quality or standards of practice are compromised. How an employee feels, thinks and behaves is moulded by the workplace and its pressing concerns of one sort or another. In effect, newcomers are invited to bond with those who've been around for a while, and that bonding behaviour is socially reinforced. If new employees have concerns about what they experience in the workplace, they are implicitly invited to attribute these to their own shortcomings or status of the novice *naïf*, not to what they see or hear (Ashforth and Anand 2003; Near and Miceli 2011).

These processes underpin the institutionalization and the normalization of wrongdoing. In their essay on how corruption becomes normalized, Ashforth and Anand (2003, p.2) defined corrupt acts as 'the misuse of authority for personal, subunit and/ or organizational gain'. This is not a criminal threshold, and these authors were considering corruption that involved cooperation between two or more people. Ashforth and Anand (2003, p.1) argued that three 'mutually reinforcing processes' – institutionalization, rationalization and socialization – underpinned what is a phased process of normalization of corruption. Institutionalization comes about when wrongdoing becomes accepted as part of a workplace culture and is carried out without thought – people adapt and become habituated to this institutionalized culture. Self-deception allows the person to believe the acts or actions are not really wrong, that others are doing it, or that the end result justifies the minor wrongdoing (Near and Miceli 2011).

Table 3.1 sets out Ashforth and Anand's (2003) phased process of normalization. In Phase 1, the initial act of wrongdoing occurs in an organizational climate that tolerates poor practice, or otherwise tacitly tolerates or ignores amoral actions. A key factor in this phase is the quality and style of leadership: laissez-faire, absent and weak leadership permits (by not intervening or stopping) the growth of corrupt or poor practice.

Table 3.1 Normalization of corrupted practice

	Phase 1	Phase 2	Phase 3
Key process	Ethical climate permits, tolerates, ignores amoral actions.	'Successful' amoral decision/ act is incorporated in organizational memory.	Corruption becomes normative, adapted to and enacted mindlessly.
Key factor	Leadership.	Subculture. Particular identities and subgroups.	Systemic momentum.

Adapted from Ashforth and Anand 2003, p.5.

Leadership is of enormous significance in modelling what is valued, above anything else, in an organization, whatever its corporate mission statements say. In Phase 1, leaders do not have to engage in corruption themselves to serve as role models; their emphasis on ends not means, their intentional or unintentional reward, condoning or turning a blind eye to poor practice is enough. Organizational structures and processes often contrive to insulate senior managers from blame, further encouraging corruption.

In Phase 2 of this model, corruption and poor practice become embedded. 'Organizational memory' – how an organization as an entity acquires, stores and uses knowledge to do its business – will store recollections of when poor practice was ignored or tacitly rewarded. An organizational assumption is born: what is not sanctioned is nevertheless acceptable. As corrupt practices are embedded, the organizational culture draws on ostensible organizational values to normalize, rationalize and then to justify the act. Otherwise decent, right-minded people may turn away from their personal values of fairness and justice, and towards the values of the corrupted culture. Fitting in and conforming to organizational norms and practices takes precedence.

In Phase 3 of Ashforth and Anand's model of how corruption becomes normalized, poor or corrupt practices are routinized, institutionalized and repeated. To increase efficiency, routines break down specialised tasks into chunks: 'The result is that individuals may perform their tasks without knowing how their individual actions, in conjunction with the actions of others, contribute to the enactment of a corrupt practice' (Ashforth and Anand 2003, p.12). Corruption or poor practice is embedded in a series of interdependent processes, and so link one person in with another. The routinization dampens down any awareness that morality, standards or decency are compromised, and group norms and the wider context reinforce this. What is routine, is taken for granted: 'Corruption thus becomes resistant not only to change, but to examination' (Ashforth and Anand 2003, p.15). It becomes an undiscussable, in other words.

Ashforth and Anand (2003) speculated that institutionalization, rationalization and socialization are each required to embed corruption. It is extremely hard for employees to uproot corruption once it has taken hold: typical ripostes ('you don't understand company culture', 'you're not one of us', 'you're not a team player') may easily silence the employee who attempts to challenge. Whistleblowers are likely to hear these accusations directed at themselves.

ETHICS AND HUMAN AGENCY

There are many paradoxes apparent in political and public reaction to scandals and outrages about failures in health and social care. A familiar refrain is the search for the person or persons *responsible* for the failure (these are inevitably frontline staff; rarely, if ever, those paid to run the organization), sitting alongside blame of individuals who knew about the wrongdoing but did not speak out (a convenient oversight, as so often professionals have spoken out and have been silenced for their trouble). The paradox is person-focused, not situation-located. It is a reaction that ignores the influence of organizational culture on individual behaviour, and indeed in leading to problems that themselves become serious failings. The paradoxical reaction is framed in the belief that human agency and free will can be exercised to counteract bad actions of the ill-intentioned. But human agency is not an entity that exists outside the social settings of a person's life: agentic capability and behaviour – the how and what the person does – are socially constructed in relationships and transactions with others, in the environment of the workplace (Bandura 2008).

For Bandura (2008), human agency has four features. First, intentionality, where people have *intention* to act in ways that align with action plans and goals in organizations. In groups, this intention is expressed as collective or shared intention. Second, agency involves *forethought*, where goals and intentions are visualized and the outcome anticipated – if A does B, then C will follow. Third, agency takes in *self-reactiveness*, involving self-regulation, and the ability to construct and follow a course of action. Fourth, and as a facet of human agency, *self-reflectiveness* allows the person to examine and reflect upon their own functioning.

In his social cognitive theory, Bandura distinguished three modes of agency – individual, proxy and collective. People don't do as they like, nor are they puppets of the situation they are in. Human functioning is ingrained in social systems: 'a product of a reciprocal interplay of intrapersonal, behavioural, and environmental determinants' (Bandura 2008, p.94). So agency is situated within a broad network of social influences and systems that guide, shape and regulate human affairs with rules, sanctions, rewards. And, of course, social systems are a product of human activity, so the circle is completed.

Moral agency pertains to a person with the ability to act or not to act, adopting standards of right and wrong: 'In the face of situational inducements to behave in inhumane ways, they can choose to resist prepotent social pressures by exerting self-influence' (Bandura 2008, p.117). In this way, moral agency can inhibit, or be proactive, while moral conduct is regulated by personal, social and legal sanctions, whose effects are mediated through cognitive processes that weigh up the anticipated risks and potential consequences. The capacity for moral agency is founded on the sense of personal identity, moral standards and behavioural regulation. People thus exercise some influence over how situations influence them, and how they shape the situations they are in.

Unethical conduct becomes more likely when people are decoupled from their cognitive control mechanisms. There are many ways of disengaging moral control: morally good people may unknowingly contribute to bad actions through disconnected subdivisions of work and diffused responsibility. Safeguards built into social systems to uphold compassionate behaviour, as well as personal moral standards, may mitigate this. The process of moral disengagement can get underway with the softening and euphemising of language to disguise bad acts:

> Cognitive restructuring of harmful conduct through moral justifications, sanitizing language, and exonerating comparisons, taken together, is the most powerful set of psychological mechanisms for disengaging moral control. Investing harmful conduct with high moral purpose not only eliminates self-censure, but it engages self-approval in the service of destructive exploits. (Bandura 1999, p.196)

So, softening up language in health and social care – for example banally presenting a decision with lifelong consequences as 'your choice', or chopping up the patient or service user experience of health and social care into chunks, each distinct and dissociated from the other, sets up conditions where otherwise moral and well-intentioned people disengage from the outcomes, those end results of their work for the people they serve.

PEOPLE ARE SOCIAL ANIMALS

As noted, fitting into the culture of a workplace team or group is often an essential criterion for appointment into most jobs in health and social care. That organization of the experience of being a team player is what Goffman (1974) called a 'frame', or set of concepts and perspectives that organize experience and guide the actions of people and groups. Shared definitions of a situation help organize social events and how people are involved in them. So if the frame is a workplace discussion, certain understandings for those involved flow from that, shaping what is appropriate to the moment, what the current reality is for those present. Once individuals share the common meaning of the frame, they can join in and play their part.

To play their part in the workplace, people interact with others. People readily form social attachments under most conditions, and put up resistance when their social bonds are threatened. Baumeister and Leary (1995, p.498) suggested the need to belong, or belongingness, may be almost as compelling as the need for food, and human culture – in this we may include workplace culture – is significantly conditioned by the pressure to achieve belongingness. A simple random allocation of people to one group and not another, without any other trait matching, may be enough for individuals to show favouritism or preference for in-group members over those in the out-groups, without knowing anything about them (Tajfel et al. 1971).

People who share common experiences, such as working together, or who are simply exposed to each other socially, tend to form friendships and attachments. Belongingness may well be a fundamental human need, especially in relation to the immediate behavioural, cognitive and emotional reactions to social acceptance and social rejection. The need to belong has a strong effect on people's cognitions, emotions and behaviours; a chronically unmet need to belong and social isolation have many profound negative impacts on a person (Gere and Macdonald 2010; Holt-Lunstad et al. 2015).

So the ability to work in a team ranks high in many lists of essential requirements for a job. Getting along with others is socially desirable. But this isn't a path to paradise. Working in groups or teams can both shift and shape individual responses, behaviours and attitudes, and not always for the best. The opinions and judgements of the group can become very fixed, and be held much more strongly than individual opinions (Moscovici and Zavalloni 1969). Groups accept higher risk levels than the individuals making up the group. The social attractiveness of belonging and being accepted into a group creates a social bubble, a cosy subculture where group difference equates to superiority, and compartmentalizes the subgroup from wider culture. Where membership is prized in these in-crowds, people can leave scruples by the door in a desire to meet their need to belong.

This all presents another paradox. Self-regulation and individual responsibility are frequently trumpeted as an antidote to poor or corrupt practice in health and social care. Duties to report wrongdoing are laid upon the person, not the health and social care organization. But life, or certainly human behaviour, is not that simple. Mead et al. (2009) looked at the influence of self-control on an individual's behaviour, as 'short-term-gain-to-be-selfish' versus 'long-term-rewards-of-being-virtuous', with all the social acceptance that may flow from that. In this, self-control meant 'the capacity to alter one's responses, such as by overriding some impulses in order to bring behaviour in line with goals and standards'. If honesty depended on self-control 'then the situational state of one's capacity for self-control' should influence how an individual responded to opportunities for cheating (Mead *et al.* 2009, p.594). In two social experiments, Mead *et al.* tested whether dishonest behaviour increased when resources for self-control had been depleted by prior exertion; they speculated that acts of self-control drew on a common resource that becomes depleted with use. They found that when self-control resources had been worn out, as it were, by prior acts of self-control, people were more likely to cheat. After one act of self-control, people performed worse than on a subsequent, unrelated self-control task: 'In effect, the moral muscle loses some of its strength' (Mead *et al.* 2009, p.594). It seems that being good and not doing harm as an individual is harder if one is the only person doing the heavy lifting. We need others to share the load.

It is not unreasonable, then, to look at how situational factors can influence the propensity of people to lie. People are more likely to lie when they are rewarded for so doing, and where there are performance pressures and rewards for achievement. When organizations place people under extreme pressure they are more likely to lie. If promotion, appraisal and financial bonuses are caught up in this, then the likelihood of lying is increased, and ethical action is diluted or evaporates (Grover and Hui 2005). The pressure on those working in health and social care services to do the best with less and keep quiet about the consequences, does not create an environment supportive of sustained ethical action, nor of speaking out about failings of care.

GROUPS: NOT ALWAYS YOUR FRIEND

Providing health or social care services to citizens is very much a team enterprise. Group work is a key building block of an organization's work, and fitting in with one's colleagues makes for an easier time at work than when unmanaged conflict runs riot. Power and personal dynamics can make working with others a pleasure or a misery. Whether pleasure or pain, groups amplify, rather than correct, perceptual distortions and errors of judgement that group members, and thence the group, hold. Group thinking and functioning can be blighted by cascade effects – that is, what others (in-crowd, powerful personalities) say or do. Groups polarize thinking. And, tellingly, groups focus on and enlarge what everybody knows anyway, rather than seeking out and paying careful attention to critical information that could be drawn upon, or that only a few people may have (Sunstein 2014). In short, people, as social animals, feel happier in the pack, but the results of that pack mentality may not be the best available.

It gets worse. Groups made up of similar people, people who adopt the same mindset, who are 'one of us', tend to buy into the prevailing orthodoxy of the group, and will develop more rigidly aligned views of their work together. When like-minded people meet regularly, without sustained exposure to competing views, their thinking becomes polarized. Two mechanisms are at play in this. First, people's beliefs and behaviours are socially influenced – what others do or think sets the frame for an individual's response. People want to maintain their reputation and self-perception, and be well thought of by those they work with. Second, are what Sunstein and Hastie (2015) called the limited 'argument pools' that exist within any group. These pools limit, or ring-fence, what group members consider, and the ways they frame their points of view. They typically screen out receiving new information, or any need to find 'unconventional' wisdom to confirm or disconfirm their existing fixed views.

Group polarization is strong and resilient, unless sustained efforts are made by people in deliberating bodies to listen and embrace views that are not corseted into a predetermined line, or 'one of us' thinking. This poses another double bind. People want to be seen favourably by others, and social comparison (that is, comparison with one's peers) moves people to adjust their position in line with dominant thinking. Within groups it seems people are likely to want to take a position of a certain socially preferred type, or align with the orthodoxy prevailing in that group. One person's position on an issue is partly a function of all arguments presented by others. The most persuasive arguments shift the group, the board, the team, in one direction, polarising the response and skewing the argument pool in one direction. People will have thought about one or some of the predictable points made, but not have access to wider arguments and ideas that challenge these and sit outside conventional thinking, and the stranglehold of 'one of us' (Sunstein and Hastie 2015).

This is not to suggest that people are biased to 'this over that' at the start, nor that they disregard evidence, although either or both may be the case. The point is narrower: people may listen to each other and consider various points of view within a narrow frame. But if the range and scope of that deliberation are limited to those predictable argument pools, and if the balance of the information in those pools supports one conclusion or reinforces the status quo, then that will hold sway. People like to get on with others. If there are enough attractive 'others', that is, people who are well regarded by others and not beyond the parameters of convention for that group, then group members will coalesce around them. When people bond and make affective ties, diversity and disagreement become sidelined and the number of divergent points of view decreases. So the argument pool narrows, and intensifies the crystallization of the social influences on choice. When people are deliberating with 'people like us', their views will be reinforced and shifted towards greater polarization (Sunstein and Hastie 2015).

For organizations, leaders and managers in health and social care, the design of institutions requires a system of checks and balances to protect against the harmful impacts of groupthink, those limited argument pools and that polarized thinking. For Sunstein and Hastie (2015), the value of deliberation as a social phenomenon depends, considerably, on social context, as well as on the nature of the process and the social relations between participants. Organizations and service systems can, of course, increase access to diverse information pools, and create space where deliberation does not insulate people from the non-likeminded. But mostly they don't. It is the whistleblower's disclosure that may expose the fault lines in these comfortable, yet narrow, information pools.

MINORITY INFLUENCE CAN MAKE A DIFFERENCE

All the foregoing may suggest there's no hope for the individual who wants to think and act ethically in the face of poor practice, and not run with the pack. While the influence of the group, group norms and the part played by power and fear whip people into line in the workplace, there is another part – more than a bit part – where the minority can influence the *zeitgeist* and the way of doing business as usual. As Serge Moscovici's (1976, 1980) work on minority influence illustrated, a consistent minority view, or sets of behaviour in a group, can shift a majority.

Minority influence, as a form of social influence resulting from exposure to a consistent minority position in a group, is generally felt only after a period of time. It tends to produce private acceptance of the views expressed by the minority. Since minority influence doesn't spring from social pressures or norms to fall into line, its power to sway is based on information, new arguments, or points of view that cause others to think again about their views. Rather like an initially ill-fitting shoe that eases up with wearing, the minority's different or discomforting views may, over time, become comfortable to a majority. For this to happen, four main influences are at play. To shift a majority view, the minority needs to be consistent, have confidence in their view, be unbiased and not have personal axes to grind and meet the challenge of not becoming brow-beaten by abuse or criticism. A minority that chops and changes its views weakens its influence capacity: holding the line and staying consistent, with confidence, makes the difference. Getting the majority to consider, discuss and debate arguments and alternatives increases the chance that the minority can shift the argument. In this, the support from others in the minority is critical to avoid individuals becoming marginalized, victimized and scapegoated. There is safety in numbers, even when those numbers may amount to no more than 1+1 (Moscovici, Lage and Naffrechoux 1969).

In his work on the Holocaust and the role of bystanders in helping Jews and persecuted minority groups escape the Nazis, Staub (1989, p.20) found that opposition from bystanders 'whether based on moral or other grounds' had the potential to change the perspectives of perpetrators and other bystanders, 'especially if the bystanders act at an early point on the continuum of destruction'. Bystanders, as witnesses to the persecution but not directly affected by it, shaped the responses of others by their own action and reactions to the Holocaust. Their non-compliance with orders and demands made on them may have delayed death in some cases, enabling people to escape. Protest, resistance, non-compliance at an early stage can prevent worse atrocities: bystanders have tremendous power to speak out and stop what's happening (Staub 1989). While there are very real reasons for people working in health and social care to keep quiet about professional concerns they have – the threats of losing one's job, income and career are not insignificant trifles – speaking out with others, and with legal or trade union advice, can transform the bystander into a whistleblower.

BAD APPLES, BAD BARRELS

When things go wrong in health and social care, lower ranking managers or frontline professionals involved may be disciplined or sacked. With the so-called bad apples removed, those basic grade staff remaining may well be put through retraining programmes, where policies are inevitably 'reviewed', and those 'lessons' re-learned once more (Ash 2013). The 'bad apple' narrative attributes unethical or poor practice to the bad behaviour of one or a few bad apples, lacking in some moral fibre, character, competence. Extending the metaphor, according to the 'bad barrel' argument something happens in the organization to make bad the otherwise 'good' apples. In this process, bad behaviour might be attributed to a lack of reinforcement of ethical behaviour. Treviño and Youngblood (1990) argued that both the apples and the barrel, both the organization and the individual are relevant, not just one or the other; behaving ethically – doing the right thing – in organizations depends on a complex interplay of individual difference, how people think about ethical decisions, and how organizations manage reward and punishment.

Zimbardo (2008) stretched the bad apple and bad barrel metaphor further, claiming that it wasn't only the bad apples and bad barrels that should hold our attention, but also the *bad barrel makers*, or the wider social, economic and political context in which organizations operate. In the UK, health and social care are public goods. If the barrel makers go bad – for example, by destroying the integrity of a national health service by selling bits of it off to global pharmaceutical companies, or by setting more and more indiscriminate targets (aptly renamed 'instruments of torture' by Toynbee, 2015) that hijack the focus and attention of those delivering health and care to citizens – then the results are felt not by performance measures presented to boards, councils or Whitehall, but by those delivering and receiving the service. A solicitor interviewed for the *Freedom to Speak Up* review (Francis 2015) nailed this:

> The protected disclosure [whistleblowing] doesn't come out of the ether. Usually it's clinicians who see that there's a problem, and it may not be something – more often than not we're not talking about individual events or surgeons where surgery goes wrong and a patient is injured in a surgery. It's more often than not, in my experience, organisational problems, very often related to funding and staffing and resources and things like that, which then has knock-on effects which means that the service that's being provided to services as patients or whatever they may be, is risky. (Vandekerckhove and Rumyantseva 2014, p.30)

The bad barrel makers corrupt the barrels, as well as the apples. The whistleblower may be the one to call out the bad barrel, and the bad barrel maker.

CULTURES ARE CRITICAL

This chapter has considered the all-encompassing influence organizational cultures of health and social care systems have on those working in them. The influence of these cultures is experienced at every level of the organization, yet largely remains unexplored within that organization, beyond the superficial, instrumental, often ill-informed statements about how important it is. Organizational straplines and symbols intended to convey a cultural message do exactly that, but not always the one intended. Deep-digging into the core of these cultures to locate and understand those 'undiscussables' is needed, bedded in as routine, everyday practice, not as a colourful conclusion to the board's annual away day. How these cultures respond to the whistleblower speaks more authentically about the organization than its public proclamations of its ethicality. Consider this from an NHS workforce director who spoke to the *Freedom to Speak Up* review:

> I think the approach that's often taken (in the NHS) is 'person A has raised some concerns; is it a protected disclosure? Not yet. Then we don't need to worry about it.' And again, I think that comes from this thing of seeing it as a litigation risk/HR issue rather than saying, 'How do we look into these concerns without having to escalate things?' (Vandekerckhove and Rumyantseva 2014, pp.18–19)

This sort of response to 'person A's' concerns does nothing to see if there really *is* a problem that needs rectification; it does nothing to assess the risk to patient safety; and it remains silent on the possibility that similar, much bigger concerns may be present elsewhere. That is the organizational culture at work.

The following chapter extends this discussion by examining strategies of silence and denial in the workplace, and the consequences for ethical practice in health and social care that a passive obedience to authority presents. This is the terrain that a whistleblower finds they are on when they raise a concern.

CHAPTER 4

SILENCE AND DEVICES OF DENIAL

Whistleblowers, as we know, may not be greeted with gratitude. The whistleblower raises concerns about harmful, dangerous, corrupt practices or behaviour. Very often what they are disclosing is known about by others, who maintain the fiction that what is happening isn't actually. Their disclosure may be ignored, denied or sidelined, as if it had never been made. This silence may be in the face of wrongdoing that is in plain sight, that others are aware of, but which is denied. There are some deep dynamics at work here which, like anaerobic bacteria that thrive without oxygen to destroy body tissue, suppurate and drain the vitality of the organization.

This chapter discusses the 'shapes and sounds' of organizational silence and denial of wrongdoing. It is in three parts. The first considers the social dynamics of silence in the workplace, and the psychology of group behaviour in maintaining that silence. Second, Milgram's work on obedience to authority is revisited. This part considers whether the findings of his work – that otherwise unremarkable, good, honest people can perpetrate harm when an authority orders them so to do – are still salient (they are). Third, devices and strategies of denial of harm and wrongdoing in the workplace are identified, and the actions and inaction of Rotherham Metropolitan Borough Council in England in tackling the systematic sexual exploitation of children and young people over many years in that locality and are examined as a case study of systemic institutionalized denial of harm.

KEEPING QUIET

At a macro level, gagging orders and confidentiality clauses in employment contracts have kept, and in some sectors still keep, wrongdoing under wraps. The interplay between confidentiality, keeping secrets, silence and speaking out is complex. Interviews with 18 nurses in Australia, each with first-hand experience of whistleblowing, illustrated how they regarded confidentiality. Two particular themes were clear for these nurses: confidentiality meant enforced silence; and confidentiality isolated and marginalized the person who was forced to maintain it in the face of wrongdoing (Jackson *et al.* 2011). In health and social care, and certainly for medical, healthcare and social care registrants, confidentiality (with some exceptions) is a professional and moral obligation. Even so, organizational confidentiality can breach ethics and legitimize secrets. Cloaked as confidentiality, this 'secret-keeping' can set in chain events that influence the culture of the organization, and which perpetuate and justify keeping ever more secrets, thereby isolating employees and creating an organizational culture where rumour and gossip flourish.

Just as speaking out about wrongdoing, poor practice or corruption has risks, so, too, does staying silent. When a person goes along with harmful organizational norms and doesn't raise concerns, that *not* speaking may lead to feelings of helplessness. Staff turnover may rocket, as people leave for other jobs where they are spared the frustration that accompanies the daily compromise of shutting up (Milliken and Morrison 2003). At its extreme, staying silent in the face of poor or corrupt practice in health or social care costs lives. Employees may want anonymous whistleblowing in the workplace, but that may be little more than an escape route with a dead end, or 'an instrumental solution to a discursive problem, the problem of not being able to talk about what we are doing' (Alford 2001, p.36). In reality, disclosure about wrongdoing can never be anonymous: an organization's first response when such a report is received is to track down who made it. Organizational silence, the not speaking out about poor practice or corrupted care, is a huge drain on those working in an organization that doesn't want to hear bad news, whatever its whistleblowing window dressing of policy and procedures.

'Silence' is non-action or inaction with many causes. Fear of being punished, of being labelled a troublemaker (too often the antonym of 'team player'), or of getting a poor performance appraisal, can all keep people quiet and close down open discussion about what's going on and why it shouldn't go on. Managers may be unskilled, unwilling or unable to give feedback to either their superiors or subordinates, about shortfalls in practice, quality or safety. Managers may implicitly discourage upward communication of information about organizational performance from employees, by not acting on it (ignore) or by dismissing the employee's concerns (shoot the messenger). The primary organizational imperative may be to control costs and meet targets, with the deadening emphasis on consensus by any means necessary. Employees are rewarded for their passive acquiescence; along with their managers, they come to believe that speaking out is not worth the effort, that voicing opinions is dangerous.

All this comes at a high price and it is not money. A homogenous health or social care workforce or workplace, staffed by people who share similar beliefs and values, delivering consistency and sameness despite the diversity of human need presented to it every day, will gradually cease to honour the value of difference, and that includes points of view critical to the 'business as usual' of the organization. Bland homogeneity stamps out diversity, debate and constructive dissent, and creates a workplace culture where speaking out against this grain becomes impossible without being socially marginalized by colleagues, or suffering sanction by employers. Organizations where silence about wrongdoing is, paradoxically, deafening, share common features. These include the strong strategic emphasis on cost control; little or no tolerance of dissent; and leadership by people with a background in economics or finance. The longer top managers stay in post in the same organization, the more homogenous top management is likely to become (in terms of race, age, gender, wealth, core values, difference from main workforce), and the stronger and more resilient the organizational cultural norms, practices and beliefs that exist around silence and shutting up (Morrison and Milliken 2000).

When employees coordinate work across an organization they are likely to talk to others about the place, and its culture and management. These conversations may well reinforce preheld views that keeping quiet about wrongdoing is the best tactic, as the organization will not be interested in hearing anything but good news. Fear of retaliation for speaking out about wrongdoing plays a significant part in keeping people quiet. Just having a policy, procedure or written code in place is unlikely to be enough to get people to speak up and speak out about wrongdoing: the organizational culture and the experience of those working in it are far more powerful (Keenan 1990). When an employee falls in line with the unspoken organizational 'rule' about keeping quiet, about not making a fuss and instead looking the other way, they are buying into organizational silence. They are acting in accord with the inauthenticity of an organizational culture that has policies, but not the practice, of speaking out.

Keeping quiet (silence) or speaking out (whistleblowing) may be on opposite ends of a spectrum of organizational behaviour, but the dynamics at play between them is more complex than a simplistic 'either/or', 'this or that'. Raising concerns in the NHS mostly happens outside formal whistleblowing policies and procedures; most concerns raised do not become protected disclosures under the UK Public Interest Disclosure Act (Jones and Kelly 2014). It is what *happens* to those concerns, and how they are responded to, that creates and reinforces an organizational culture of silence. Even amidst all the chatter and noise of an organization, the upshot of not acting on concerns, of ignoring or marginalizing those who raise them, is still 'silence'.

THE SOUND OF SILENCE

Results of the 2014 Roffey Park (a UK management and leadership centre) management survey of 1400 managers and 200 other employees across different organizations and sectors, did not paint a hopeful picture of the ethical climate of those private and public sector organizations. Half of those surveyed had observed misconduct; one-third did not report it, mostly because they did not think anything would be done about it, or because they believed they would suffer reprisal if they did. They were more likely to walk than to talk. One in five of respondents did not expect their organization to treat people fairly; this lack of trust and avoidance of accountability were seen as the key blocks to organizational development and change. And four out of ten said there was a disconnect between the public values of the company and its real-time behaviour towards its employees and its business (Lucy, Poorkavoos and Wellbelove 2014).

It is not the case that employees in workplaces where wrongdoing is tolerated do not speak about what it is that is tolerated. In a cacophony of moaning or blaming in the workplace, the sound of silence is screened out. *Contexts* to organizational silence are where its causes, forms and meaning are located; they are crucial for understanding the meaning and significance of keeping quiet (Pinder and Harlos 2001). These contexts, or surroundings, include power relations, dominance, hierarchy and authority. Cultures of injustice develop, characterized by the suppression of conflict, a valuing of job relations over human relations, and an emphasis on production through competitive individualism. 'Deaf ear syndrome' (Peirce, Smolinski and Rosen 1998) discourages employees' direct and open expression of discontent.

If silence is understood as a response to injustice, it becomes a form of communication. Pinder and Harlos distinguished between quiescent and acquiescent silence. Employee quiescence was silence by *omission*, or suffering in silence. Employee acquiescence, on the other hand, involved *submission* or condoning. Acquiescent employees were less conscious of their silence, less ready or willing to change than their quiescent counterparts, and they gave up hope of bringing about change by their resignation and tacit acceptance of the status quo. Quiescent employees were, though, more aware that there were alternatives, that wrongdoing was not unchangeable or irreversible, that things could be changed. The dissonance they experienced from this double bind (knowing change was possible yet feeling powerless to bring it about) led to more stress, with emotions of fear, anger, despair and cynicism dominating (Pinder and Harlos 2001). It is whistleblowers who act to break through the double bind when they raise the concerns that acquiescent others do not.

SPIRAL OF SILENCE

People are more likely to speak up if they think their position is supported by others, and they stay quiet when they believe it is not. Organizational voice – speaking up, speaking out about something – is influenced by individual perceptions of the attitudes towards the issue within their workgroup (Bowen and Blackmon 2003). A 'spiral of silence' can explain how dominant opinions form over time (Noelle-Neumann 1974). Spirals of silence restrict openness of discussion; threats of social isolation, or the fear of it, keep people quiet. The willingness of people to express a view or to speak out is influenced by personal opinions and the external environment (their perceptions of what others think or would do), as well as what they perceive to be prevailing climate of opinion.

This spiral of silence is especially powerful when there is potential for social isolation within a workgroup. Homogenous groups tend to similar opinions: people in them know, or think they know, the same things; they may communicate freely but within the pre-formed, implicitly understood boundaries of group opinions and beliefs. Where individuals in a minority fear they will be marginalized if they speak freely, they are less likely to speak out. To keep the sense of social cohesion in the group, out-groups are under pressure to assimilate. Those in power have little incentive to adjust their behaviour to accommodate other groups; minority groups are under counter-pressure to assimilate to avoid being socially isolated. These spirals of silence show how people's opinions about issues are not fixed, but change in response to local and external opinions (Bowen and Blackmon 2003).

BLACK SHEEP AND WALLS OF SILENCE

Staying silent in the face of wrongdoing has its pay-offs, beyond the crude 'wanting to fit in' with one's team mates. 'Black sheep' is Muehlheusser and Roider's (2008) description for those who do wrong in the workplace. Their honest (or non-wrongdoing) workmates don't report this and so set up a 'wall of silence', which has an equilibrium: the black sheep misbehave and honest members set up the wall of silence. The honest members do this because they do not want to lose benefits from cooperating with black sheep in the future – they may have to call in a favour down the line, so the wall of silence puts some credit in the bank. Muehlheusser and Roider speculated that this was more likely in asymmetric teams, where the benefit from cooperation was greater for honest members than for the black sheep. There are substantial benefits in the workplace from being an accepted group member, for example, back-up and cooperation from colleagues in tricky situations – and the impetus to ensure future cooperation maintains the wall of silence. Keeping this wall in place is a conspiratorial buy-in, 'where a group of people tacitly agree to outwardly ignore something of which they are personally aware' (Zerubavel 2006, p.2).

Conspiracies of silence, keeping quiet, not rocking the boat and the absence of hope that anything will change, are all reasons why people don't speak up about what they see, hear or sense is wrong. Dread of being labelled as troublemaker or moaner, fear of loss of trust, respect and relationship, of retaliation, punishment, loss of job, and feelings of futility are all reasons those keeping quiet have given for their silence. These all reside in the basic requirement of the workplace that employees obey rules, directives and authority.

OBEDIENCE TO AUTHORITY

Stanley Milgram's studies of obedience were landmark pieces of 20th-century social science (Milgram 1974). Films and TV programmes on the findings regularly appear (e.g., the 2009 BBC2 TV *Horizon* programme 'How violent are you?'; the 2015 film *Experimenter*). In his original experiments, Milgram recruited volunteers in what they were told was an experiment to help people learn. Those supposedly 'learning' were actors. The volunteers were encouraged by scientists in white coats (also actors, and also in on the experiment's true purpose) to administer what they were told were increasingly powerful electric shocks to the 'learners' if they failed to answer a question correctly.

The finding of these experiments that has entered the public imagination was the passive willingness of ordinary, otherwise well-adjusted human beings – the volunteers – to inflict what so-called 'men in white coats' (people in authority) told them were electric shocks that, had they been real not fake, could have caused serious harm, or possibly death.

The ethics of Milgram's experiments have been debated and contested for decades. The legacy of the findings – that perfectly ordinary people, who aren't psychopaths, deviants, abusers, otherwise disordered or violent men and women, when calmly ordered by an authority to perform a blatantly harmful and possibly deadly act, are likely to obey the order – is sobering. Today, researchers wanting to replicate Milgram's work, as Milgram set it up, would be refused permission by ethics committees. Be that as it may, understanding whether and how ethical mores and social pressures to obey an 'authority' change over time remains central to any attempt to appreciate why people don't speak out when they are asked to do something they fear will harm another.

Half a century after Milgram's work, Burger (2009) secured ethical approval to replicate a part of one of Milgram's experiments. Burger did this by protecting the wellbeing of the volunteers, who had been led to believe they were administering electric shocks of increasing intensity to learners. In Milgram's experiment, almost eight out of ten volunteers continued past the 150 volts point, which was when the learner/actor started to protest verbally and ask for the shocks to stop. When this happened, in both Milgram's and Burger's experiments, the eponymous 'man in a white coat' (*sic*) supposedly in charge of the experiment, quietly encouraged the volunteer to continue. The vast majority – 79 per cent of Milgram's subjects – went past the 150 volts point. Obedience rates in Burger's experiment were only slightly lower than in Milgram's. In Burger's study, volunteers who saw a confederate (someone in on the experiment and also pretending) disobey the experimenter's instruction to keep going, obeyed as often as those who didn't; so seeing someone else opt out did not lead the volunteer to do the same. Men and women did not behave differently in either the Milgram or Burger experiments. What did have a bearing on how likely it was that a volunteer kept on administering electric shocks was two-fold: first, their empathic concern for others (the greater their empathy, the more likely they were to refuse to continue); and second, their desire for control (the higher the desire to control, the more likely the person was to carry on with the experiment). Burger's experiment showed that attitudes to authority and obedience were little changed since Milgram's experiments over 50 years earlier.

If it's hard to spot who will obey or not obey, then the situational dimensions of that behaviour, rather than personal characteristics like gender, age or education, probably tell us more about what is going on when good people do nothing in the face of wrongdoing. In this, Bocchiaro *et al.* (2012) found much the same as Milgram and Burger. The study by Bocchiaro *et al.* involved 96 female and 53 male students ($n = 149$) with a mean age of 20.8 years. These students were asked to do something unethical by the stern, white-coated authority figure, and given the options to obey, disobey or whistleblow. All the students believed the fabricated cover story. The majority – 77 per cent – obeyed the instruction to carry out the unethical request. The minority that did not obey was split between those who simply disobeyed, and the minority of the minority who reported the unethical request to a higher authority: in other words they spoke up, spoke out, and were identified as whistleblowers. The researchers found no significant differences in personal characteristics, such as gender or religious affiliation between the different responses.

As part of this same study, people in an independent sample ($n = 138$) were asked to predict their own behaviour given the same scenario. In this component of the study, only four per cent *thought* they would obey the authority (77 per cent had actually obeyed in the main experiment, showing the scale of self-deception in underestimating personal submissiveness). None of the standard assessments of individual personality differences could usefully predict and distinguish among those who obeyed, disobeyed or whistleblew; instead, strong situational forces – what was happening to people in the situation they found themselves in – were at work, and operated on they way they behaved (Bocchiaro *et al.* 2012).

Bocchiaro and his colleagues highlighted that what we say and think we would do in a situation is not a good predictor of how we are actually likely to behave. People obeying an immoral instruction explicitly justify their morally wrong behaviour by allocating responsibility to external forces: they were just 'obeying orders', or variations on the miscreant's defence of 'he made me do it', 'it was her fault, not mine'. In other words, pinning the rap on something or somebody else is used to abdicate personal responsibility for wrongdoing. Those few who defied the immoral instruction in Bocchiaro and colleagues' experiment regarded themselves as responsible for their own actions or inactions.

So people overestimate their own ethicality, morality, capacity to act and speak out when confronted with wrongdoing. We believe we are more moral than we are. We signal virtue, but may behave dishonourably. We think we're different from our less than moral counterparts, but we are not, by and large. Behaving morally seems to be hard for people. When confronted with an unjust demand the question isn't whether to obey, but which authority to obey. Conscience? Employer? Code of practice? Client? These are not synonymous, equivalent or mutually exclusive: each is at play in the moment.

DENIAL

In the language of a psychotherapist, denial may be regarded as an unconscious defence mechanism for coping with guilt and anxiety or the need to avoid pain. Stan Cohen (a sociologist who said he thought like a psychologist) reflected on what people did with their knowledge of the suffering of others, and also what this knowledge did to the person. A common thread in states of denial is that people, organizations and societies have information that is too disturbing, threatening or anomalous to be fully absorbed and so, as a result, it is pushed away, disavowed, repressed, reinterpreted, repackaged. 'Knowing' something may be ambiguous; we are not quite conscious of what we're looking at; we know, yet don't know. Ramped up to an industrial scale, state denial occurs when powerful groups ignore injustice around them, claiming not to know what is known to others. (Cohen 2001).

Denial may look like passivity and silence, or obliviousness, apathy and indifference, but these are not the same. We can feel and care passionately about something and yet remain silent. We can believe we are speaking out but, as in childhood nightmares, our words or screams are not heard. Cohen (2001) suggested that denial was characterized by thoughts and feelings that included cognition (not facing facts); emotion (not feeling); moral emptiness (not recognizing the ethical); and action that was not right action (not tackling the wrongdoing). Types or artefacts of denial take in the bland and unremarkable, from a dulled or passive tolerance of harm, to its normalization, accommodation, acceptance or perpetration. These are socially reinforced responses. Few get chastised *at the time* for going along with the crowd, for not speaking out, or for looking the other way; denial is not a stable personality quirk that can somehow be screened out at recruitment and section, or trained or performance managed out of a workforce. (Rare would be the organization that authentically strove to root out denial, whether personal or institutional). Even if they could, organizations would likely have too much invested in maintaining denial. Careful management of organizational storylines is needed to sustain collective blindness and inconvenient truths (or convenient lies) – for example, that those in charge did not know; that a tragedy was an unfortunate, one-off local problem. If they are not informed, they do not need to turn a blind eye, as 'there is nothing to not-know' (Cohen 2001, p.68). Denial and its normalization come to reflect 'personal and cultural states in which suffering is not acknowledged' (Cohen 2001, p.52). In this, neutralization of the truth is one of denial's most powerful weapons.

STRATEGIES OF DENIAL

'Neutralization' is a strategy of denial. By neutralizing, wrongdoing is not justified but the meanings attached to it are disputed, and culpability and moral blame are evaded. Neutralizing can involve denial of responsibility: the wrongdoing was an accident; the person didn't mean to; they can't remember. Second, denial of injury makes light, or makes a joke of, the wrongdoing: it was just 'borrowing', a 'bit of fun', 'not serious'. Third, victim-blaming neutralizes by denial:

it was her fault, he is oversensitive or overreacting, a basket-case, you can't believe her, and so on. Fourth, those raising concerns are neutralized as hypocrites, liars, revenge-seekers. Fifth, neutralization can involve appeal to some higher group loyalty – the family, the team, the cause. Cohen (2001) also recognized neutralization in denial of knowledge of the wrongdoing and, insidiously, in moral indifference – saying there's nothing to neutralize. No problem. No worries.

Ignoring and blind-eyeing are like the behaviour of a child who closes her eyes to make a scary monster disappear. Such 'determined ignorance' (Cohen 2001, p.86) means what is not accepted, ceases to exist. Pressures to conform are given as reasons for inaction or harmful action – everyone was doing it; if you were there, you'd do the same. Claims of moral balance – of good and bad – are used to justify bad because some good was done. Rotherham Metropolitan Borough Council in England, discussed below, in its collective denial of the scale of child exploitation in its borough, made much of the council's winning awards for this or that, as if the investment of time and cash in winning window dressings made up for failure to protect vulnerable children and young people from sexual exploitation over many years (Casey Report 2015).

The term 'doubling' (Lifton 1986) describes the dreadful behaviour of a person in one place or part of life, then leaving that place to become 'decent' elsewhere. It is a type of split-world behaviour; the internalization and existence within one person of the 'good cop, bad cop' double act of crime fiction. For Cohen, late modern cultures reward this splitting, dissociation and numbing. 'Institutionalized hypocrisy' gets praised as 'tolerance', or real-world common sense (Cohen 2001, p.94). Means and ends are decoupled; fragmentary tasks, seemingly innocuous in themselves, add up to significant harm. The whole is greater than the sum of the parts. Such cultures of denial 'encourage turning a collective blind eye, leaving horrors unexamined or normalized as being part of the rhythms of everyday life' (Cohen 2011, p.101).

Popular slogans of the bystander not acting to stop harm – 'the truth is somewhere in between', 'I don't want to get involved', 'I want to remain neutral', 'it's nothing to do with me' – are all superficially defensible, yet deadly, denials of wrongdoing – what Cohen called 'vocabularies of exoneration' (Cohen 2001, p.76). These trite tropes litter the defence offered up by organizations where great harm has been visited upon those least able to defend themselves from it. The actions and inaction of Rotherham Metropolitan Borough Council in England to tackle the organized sexual exploitation of children and young people over many years, and in the face of evidence that was in plain sight, drew on many of these vocabularies of exoneration.

DOUBLESPEAK AND DENIAL: ROTHERHAM, ENGLAND

In February 2015, the Department for Communities and Local Government in England published an inspection report (Casey Report 2015) of Rotherham Metropolitan Borough Council, a local authority in South Yorkshire, England. This inspection followed publication in 2014 of the Jay Report on the child sexual exploitation of at least 1400 children, mainly girls, in that borough between 1997 and 2013 (Jay Report 2014). In over one-third of cases, children affected by sexual exploitation had been known to services because of child protection issues and neglect.

The inspection report resulted in the council being put on special measures, meaning its councillors were replaced by commissioners sent in by central government. The Casey Report said the council lacked leadership, the capacity to understand, accept and learn from its failure to protect vulnerable young people. It found a council '…in denial. They denied that there had been a problem, or if there had been, that it was as big as was said. If there was a problem they certainly were not told…' (Casey Report 2015, p.5). The inspectors came to the view that Rotherham Metropolitan Borough Council had 'a culture of suppressing bad news and ignoring difficult issues. This culture is deep-rooted…[the council went] to some length to cover up information and to silence whistle-blowers' (Casey Report 2015, p.11).

The actions, inactions and failures of Rotherham Metropolitan Borough Council to protect children from sexual exploitation was denial on a vast scale, and over many years. Denial, as discussed, has many faces. It may manifest as 'it's not happening', the flat refusal to acknowledge harm, wrongdoing, corruption. Denial may involve discrediting the source, blaming the messenger for the bad news. Or, in an Orwellian flourish, it may acknowledge wrongdoing but rename or reframe it as something else. Denial may involve the duplicity of acknowledging wrongdoing *but with justification*: bad *x* was necessary to counter the even worse *y*, and yes, bad things happen. Lessons have been learned.

Table 4.1, which summarizes some findings from both the 2014 Jay Report and the 2015 Casey Report on Rotherham Metropolitan Borough Council, identifies six common devices of denial that Rotherham Metropolitan Borough Council deployed. First was the straightforward refusal to acknowledge – it's not happening. In this, Rotherham drew on pretty much every device in the denial manual. It underplayed the scale of the problem. It criticized the accuracy and conclusions of rigorous research without providing any evidence of alleged flaws. The council suppressed reports. It claimed that while there might have been a problem once, things were better now, and that saying otherwise simply wasn't fair.

In the second denial device, the ever popular 'shoot the messenger', Rotherham blamed and discredited the sources for providing clear evidence that young people and children were being sexually exploited. The council treated young people with contempt by ignoring their exploitation; it claimed that the news media taking an interest in the story were 'out to get' the council and – in a curious inversion of reality – that it was they, the council, who were the victims.

The third denial was the window dressing of policies, procedures, presentations to conferences, and submissions for care awards. Work on these devoured council resources, time and money, but did little, if anything, to concertedly get to grips with the systematic, organized rape and sexual exploitation of vulnerable youngsters by older men paying for sex with minors, over many years and in many locales. The council's were displacement activities and substitutes for action.

Table 4.1 Devices of denial: Rotherham Metropolitan Borough Council, England

Devices of denial	Jay Report 2014 Findings	Casey Report 2015 Findings
1. 'It's not happening.' Refusal to acknowledge.	The scale and seriousness of CSE (child sexual exploitation) was underplayed by senior social care managers. *De facto* suppression of the draft Home Office Report 2002[1] report on child sexual exploitation because some senior officers did not believe the data it contained.	Denial: • of the accuracy of the Jay Report 2014 methods and findings • of the nature, extent and scale of CSE • of culpability, and belief that CSE was 'being dealt with elsewhere' • that CSE remained a significant problem, although acknowledging that it may have been in the past.
2. Discredit the source. Blame the messenger.	Operationally, the police gave no priority to CSE, regarded many child victims with contempt, and failed to act on their abuse as a crime.	'The media were out to get them.' Rather than considering what led to media attention, the council portrayed negative attention as politically motivated and unevidenced.
3. Window dressing and false comfort.	False assurance taken from the existence of policies and reports, without interrogation of what, if anything, they did to address organized CSE.	The council held conferences on CSE, gave papers at national forums, and entered for awards. Yet they refused to acknowledge either the nature or the scale of what was going on. Misplaced priorities: the council put resources into pursuing awards at the cost of sorting out the basics.
4. Doublespeak.	Majority of perpetrators were described as 'Asian' by victims, yet councillors did not engage directly with the Pakistani-heritage community. Staff nervousness about identifying perpetrators' ethnic origin for fear of being labelled racist. Staff remembered clear direction from their managers not to mention alleged perpetrators' ethnicity.	Alleged perpetrators were usually described as being Pakistani-heritage men. A social worker recalled a strategy meeting about an exploited young person where Pakistani-heritage taxi drivers were referred to as *'men of a certain ethnicity, engaged in a particular occupation'.* *'You couldn't bring up race issues in meetings…or you would be branded a racist.'*

5. Focus on process not outcomes.	Poor management – focus on paperwork not outcomes. The Rotherham Safeguarding Children Board developed good inter-agency policies and procedures, but rarely checked whether these were being implemented, or whether they were working.	Meetings and action plans were numerous but unproductive. The tendency was towards inertia.
6. Blame, bully, no bad news.	A chapter of a draft report on CSE (The Home Office Report 2002) severely criticized CSE agencies in Rotherham on many counts: • their alleged indifference and ignorance about CSE by managers • blaming the young people and not taking action against suspected abusers • senior police and council officers unsubstantiated claims that evidenced facts were fabricated or exaggerated. Until 2009, the prevailing culture at the most senior level of the council was bullying and 'macho'; a hostile climate in which to confront rape and CSE.	Sexist, bullying or intimidating behaviour. Fear of repercussions for speaking out. Staff spoke of being told to keep quiet, to cover up, and of a culture where 'if you want to keep your job, you keep your head down and your mouth shut.' Whistleblowers said they were marginalized, bullied, harassed and victimized as a result of raising concerns. Bad news was not welcome and difficult matters were taken off council agendas.

1 This draft Home Office report 2002 was never published. The Jay Report confirmed that 'much of what was contained in this report, and in particular the criticisms and concerns of the research officer, has been confirmed by the Inquiry from other sources' (Jay Report 2014, p.87).

Fourth, 'doublespeak denial' precluded the use of available intelligence, interrogating it with intelligence, and taking action against the perpetrators. The Pakistani heritage of most alleged perpetrators was an unmentionable fact for people who were in a position to do something, for fear of their being labelled racist, or of inciting aggression and civil disturbance from neo-fascist, far right, white supremacist groups. This was a hideous betrayal of children who were trapped in organized sexual exploitation by men old enough to be their father or grandfather.

In denial device five, managers proliferated policies and papers and multiplied meetings – busy work that was constantly exhausting, yet which privileged process over outcome, that is, taking right action for the children and young people who were raped, drugged, assaulted and sold for sex. The sixth denial was fastened into a sexist, bullying, blame culture where truth could not speak its name and bad news was sidelined. Speaking out ran counter to the council's cultural *modus operandi* that marginalized and bullied whistleblowers, and sent out the message that to keep one's job meant keeping one's mouth shut. Children and young people were blamed for being raped or trafficked, with little or no action taken against their suspected abusers.

Silence, uncritical obedience to authority and denial are the unwritten rules of organizational engagement that the whistleblower breaks. Whistleblowing so often means going against the grain of those covert, subtle (although sometimes blatant) social and professional mores of the workplace, profession or service, to stand up, rather than stand by. It is the whistleblower who calls out these devices of denial. In the next chapter, the silence of the bystander who witnesses harm but does nothing is considered, along with various strategies of self-deception. These self-deception strategies are the evil twin to the devices of denial exemplified in the failures of Rotherham Metropolitan Borough Council to protect children and young people from the lifelong consequences of prolonged sexual exploitation.

CHAPTER 5

BYSTANDERS, BLEACH AND BLIND SPOTS

For every whistleblower, there are many more who stood aside, or walked away from the problem. Circumstances, and the organizational cultures people work in, may exert pressure on a person to remain silent. This chapter looks at the social phenomenon that is 'bystanding', that is, where people in a group are less likely to step up to help out, or speak out, than a person acting alone. It considers the self-deception involved, as ethical behaviour in an organization or workplace becomes compromised – bleached out – on the slippery slope that is the tacit tolerance of poor, harmful or criminal practice; that is, until the whistleblower raises concerns. This self-deception is fuelled by the propensity of many of us to overestimate our personal ethicality and morality.

This perception bias – the tenaciously held belief that we're more moral than we mostly are – is a personal blind spot that shuts off acting to raise concerns where others have not. Personal blind spots are both magnified and mirrored in organizational blind spots, or the denial and refusal to face up and face into organizational problems that seriously compromise the quality of health or social care provided to people using those services. Not tackling these blind spots, and not paying attention to small as well as significant 'failures' of health and social care – a form of systemic attention deficit disorder, it is suggested – can have fatal consequences. The chapter revisits the disaster that was healthcare provided in Mid Staffordshire NHS Foundation Trust between 2005 and 2009. The way NHS managers and the Board there used information they had about performance (and failure) is contrasted with the use of failure data in the airline industry. Noticing the blind spots and getting wise to self-deception requires detached interrogation of things that are wrong, devoid of the blame, punishment and victimization that are so often visited upon the whistleblower who speaks out.

BYSTANDERS AND THE AVERSION OF THE GAZE

Up until the point when they speak out, whistleblowers may have been bystanders to wrongdoing. Bystanders are people who see, hear, sense or know harm or corruption is happening, but do not act to stop the wrongdoing. Wrapped up in the term 'bystander' are judgements about the person's passivity and failure to act. There are no distinguishing features or patterns of behaviour of people who are bystanders, any more than there are of those who whistleblow. It is the context or situation within which wrongdoing of some sort or another occurs, that is key.

Not intervening to stop harm – bystanding – is more likely in certain circumstances. First, when responsibilities are scattered or spread about, the 'it's not my job' defence for action (or failure to act) is more likely to be heard. Second, if a bystander has little affinity or identification with the victim, they are less likely to draw attention to harm or wrongdoing the victim suffers. Third, if people don't know what to do to draw attention to a problem, they are more likely to walk on by. Fourth, if the scale of what is wrong is simply overwhelming or beyond understanding, then the response may well be to do nothing, or simply look away (Dozier and Miceli 1985).

In their classic study of bystander non-intervention, Latané and Darley (1968) found that the likelihood of a bystander offering help was inversely related to the number of bystanders: the more people witnessing, the less likely it was that any one of them would step forward to help. Personality attributes, background measures such as education, social class or income, did not predict whether someone came to help; only the *number* of other witnesses did (Darley and Latané 1968).

This is a sobering conclusion to reach about the capacity of human beings to step out of line and speak up when harm or crime is being perpetrated. The lone whistleblower has to counter both social conditioning and group pressure to keep quiet and to conform, which are inherent in the situation that others have turned away from. If one person gets off their bystander backside, so to speak, whether for moral reasons or a simple human sense of outrage at injustice, then they can influence, and change, the perspective of others. If one person speaks out – acts – early enough, before they and others become inured to what is happening, they can, as discussed earlier, make a difference for the better (Staub 1999). Yet, paradoxically, the inaction of the do-nothing, turn-away bystander can determine the outcome of the situation the whistleblower speaks out about. It is telling that when others who know about the wrongdoing don't stand up to speak out in solidarity, whistleblowers usually lose when they raise concerns (Rothschild and Miethe 1999).

People paid to work in health and social care services are hardly bystanders, in the sense of being some random presence passively observing poor practice. (A 'random presence', the person in the street, is unlikely to pick up on dangerous or corrupt practice in health or social care unless it is unambiguously and visibly awful). What does it take for someone else to become involved in a whistleblowing matter? Latané and Darley's (1968) work on group pressures and bystander intervention suggested there were a series of steps that 'bystanders' (these were not people paid to uphold standards of public service, but chance witnesses) went through before they stopped standing by and started standing up. First, the bystander has to become aware of the problem, and decide that it is an emergency. Next the bystander has to decide they are responsible for doing something, and they must then choose a method of help or intervention, before finally acting.

The whistleblower and the act of whistleblowing illustrate some of these steps. The whistleblower is aware of the problem; others may or may not be aware. Situations of harm or corruption are serious but may not constitute an emergency at the beginning. 'Hidden' abuse that many were aware of, such as that perpetrated on people with learning disabilities at Winterbourne View in England between 2007 and 2013, for example, was not construed as an emergency, despite the frequent emergency visits people living in that place made to the local hospital. Then, once aware and concerned enough to speak out, the whistleblower has to take responsibility for raising concerns, for deciding who to take the concern to, and for deciding what form of disclosure or report to make – that is, whether through whistleblowing policies and procedures, or using other means. In the case of Winterbourne View, disclosures were not made under the UK whistleblowing law, PIDA. Whistleblower action in many ways parallels the steps Latané and Darley (1968) set out (see also Dozier and Miceli 1985). The whistleblower engages in a process of coming to speak out. But that process can become corrupted, if self-deception is strong enough to distort the whistleblower's perceptions of what they see or know.

SELF-DECEPTION, THE SLIPPERY SLOPE AND ETHICAL DEGRADATION

Alford (2001) had this to say about organizations:

> Organizations are not just undemocratic. Organizations are the enemy of individual morality. Individuals who depend on these organizations for their livelihoods may become democrats in their communities in their off-hours, but there will always be something false and partial about it. Large organizations, private and public alike, don't just control the political agenda. They are the political world that matters most to people's lives, and that part of politics that controls your career, your pay check, your health insurance, your mortgage, your retirement, and your family's economic security. Until there is room for the ethical individual in these organizations – until, that is, there is ethical commerce between the organization and civic society – the associations that make up civil society have the quality of a hobby. (Alford 2001, p.35)

This dystopian view of the morality of organizational life is unlikely to be one that many leaders or managers would publicly agree with, although privately they might. In it, Alford captures the all-enveloping hold the organization has on the lives of those who work in it, the compartmentalized nature of civic and organizational life, and the splitting of personal ethics from the exigencies of the work. Overlaying that are a number of self-deceptions that organizational psychologists and other observers have identified over decades.

Self-deception, in the context of raising concerns and whistleblowing, describes behaving in a self-interested way while, at the same time, falsely believing that moral principles are being upheld. Tenbrunsel and Messick (2004, p.233) likened such self-deception to an 'ethical bleach' that removed or stripped out the ethical colours and shades of a situation, erasing the path to taking ethical, right action. In the workplace, people typically respond to real-time pressures, workplace norms and workarounds, past practices, pressures and dilemmas, overwork, all of which leave little room (often time just to think) for any ethical examination of how work is being done to achieve expected outcomes. 'Ethical fading' – why people behave differently in actuality from what they predict they will do – is the upshot of this bleaching, in a 'process by which, consciously or subconsciously, the moral colors of an ethical decision fade into bleached hues that are void of moral implications' (Tenbrunsel and Messick 2004, p.224).

Such self-deception lies at the heart of unethical decision making and action, those small, everyday compromises and adjustments made in organizational life that, cumulatively, may amount to ethical degradation and compromise of ethical expectations at work. Self-deception fades out the moral implications of decisions; it allows people to behave incomprehensibly, at least from an outsider's vantage point. People simply may not see what is all around them. Avoiding or disguising the moral implications of decisions allows people to behave in a self-interested way, yet still believe they are acting ethically. Salvation through self-deception, but at a price.

Various devices, or enablers, drive this self-deception. They include euphemisms or softening-up leadership language like 'we take this very seriously' meaning 'we will nail whoever blew the gaff on this'. They involve slippery-slope decision making, where small, gradual adjustments – downwards – of standards and expectations occur. These are so subtle they often pass unnoticed. Or they may include errors of perception in simply not seeing or hearing what is happening – those blind eyes and deaf ears. These enablers do not feature a great deal in training on ethics in organizations, the limitations of which are discussed below (Tenbrunsel and Messick 2004).

The 'slippery slope effect' is pernicious. It psychologically anaesthetizes, so that an individual becomes inured to what is happening because they do it, see it or hear it so often. And when something becomes routine and everyday and ordinary, people stop noticing. Our perceptual biases and ways of processing vast quantities of sensory information, second by second, mean we may fail to notice ethical erosion and corrosion when that is happening slowly and incrementally. Ethical degradation on this slippery slope occurs outside the person's awareness of intentionality, or of the cause and effect of those small adjustments downwards (Gino and Bazerman 2009). People new to an organization may well pick this up, where others already in the situation have become habituated to the ethical degradation. But the newcomer's capacity to speak out will be constrained by their 'newness', by their need to fit in and get on with the job.

EXERCISING THE MORAL MUSCLE

Few people set out to wilfully and knowingly do harm to others. Ethical lapses are more likely where professional goals are compromised, as they may be in health and social care when staffing and cash are cut. As a condition of registration, and thus permission to work, UK registered medical, health and social care practitioners are required to put the wellbeing, health and care of the individual at the forefront of what they do. When organizational resourcing, practices, deficits and the like get in the way of this, talking to an employer about the impact of these shortfalls on the quality of health and social care provided – which would provide invaluable intelligence to stave off a major problem – may well backfire on the whistleblower, to the detriment, and sometimes the ending, of their otherwise unblemished career.

Dr David Drew and Dr Raj Mattu, two consultant doctors in different hospitals in the English Midlands, found this to their cost (Drew 2014; Smith 2014). Both were consultant doctors, in different specialisms, who raised concerns about practice they considered dangerous. In noticing and acting, Drew and Mattu (their individual cases and circumstances as whistleblowers are discussed later) were exceptions to the general finding that when we do the same thing over and over, it becomes automatic and then is no longer noticed. If we go along with that one 'bad' thing, we are more likely to go along with another, as we have compromised our ethical credentials: saying 'no' to the next big bad thing is harder when we have said 'yes' to a smaller one (Moore and Loewenstein 2004). That 'moral muscle' (Mead *et al.* 2009) needs regular exercise, and without this, it loses its strength to challenge wrongdoing.

WE THINK WE'RE MORE MORAL THAN WE MOSTLY ARE

The moral outrage that is political or public reaction to wrongdoing and scandal in health and social care pretty much always ends up with statements, commitments and calls for 'this must never happen again'. This scandalized shock is perched on a misplaced sense of the ethical rightness of our own behaviour. Sad to say, people generally overestimate their own goodness. People want to see themselves as moral, competent, and deserving (Chugh, Bazerman and Banaji 2005). We narrate our stories and we believe them. We avoid the secrets that we keep to ourselves, yet we claim objectivity. We believe our own judgements are less prone to bias than those of others. Our judgements about ourselves, about others and the rightness of ethical behaviour, are clouded by numerous cognitive and motivational biases. We rate ourselves as above average (a statistically unlikely feat) on valued social domains such as doing right and being good, and we conclude that we are more moral than we mostly are. When evaluating past behaviour, we believe we behaved more ethically than we actually did (Ehrlinger, Gilovich and Ross 2005; Tenbrunsel *et al.* 2010).

So self-deception extends to biased perceptions that people (we) hold about their (our) own ethicality. People claim that they do, and will, behave more ethically than actually happens in practice. We favour self-seeking interpretations and accounts; the ethical decisions we make may be biased as a result of our inclination to see ourselves this way, and may lead to behaviours that contradict what we *say* we do. We want to see ourselves as moral, competent and deserving (Tenbrunsel *et al.* 2010). This capacity for self-deception will override the message of any ethics training that organizations periodically deliver to staff, and the requirements of professional codes and statutory standards placed on registered health and social care professionals.

Much unethical behaviour occurs outside conscious awareness. This is not a characteristic of overtly unethical people, but rather of all of us. Unethical behaviour is rooted in the ordinary. To understand and change the ethicality of human action we need to go beyond the common assumption that ethical lapses are the result of people choosing a bad thing over a good one (that is, what is right) (Bazerman and Banaji 2004). The glamorous illusion that is free will tempts human beings into claiming responsibility and intention for things over which they have little or no control (Wegner 2002). Traditional approaches to ethics training and education about ethics are based on this fallacious belief that people easily recognize the ethical and moral dimensions of everyday actions. The more familiar, the more everyday the decision or action, the less likely that its moral aspects will be considered at all (Bazerman and Tenbrunsel 2012). The results of ethics training are short-lived. Training is mostly narrow in focus, often using case studies that ask trainees to focus on the moral aspects of a decision. Inevitably, they choose the high moral road: they are in the training room, in a peer group, with its own pressures to signal virtue and be seen to be worthy, moral and upright. 'Big questions' about ethical dilemmas asked of respondents, such as 'would you shelter a Jewish child from the Nazis?' just won't – ever – be faced by most folk (Alford 2001). Twenty-first century MBA students are unlikely – ever – to be asked to put their own life, or that of anyone close to them, on the line for their beliefs. But whistleblowing on problems in the workplace will much more likely put the employee in a position of risking their livelihood, their way of life, their relationships, family, sense of self and the goodness of others. There is little, if any, discussion in professional training or in the outputs of the myriad regulators, that is much good in preparing people for, *de facto*, becoming a scapegoat.

That is not surprising. This 'goodness training' on ethics and ethical decision making may well not survive career pressures. These include not upsetting those who have power over the development of that career. Medicine and medical training are a case in point. Goldie and his colleagues (2003) looked at the attitudes and potential whistleblowing behaviour of medical school students in Glasgow, Scotland, by administering the Vignette of the Ethics in Health Care Instrument before and after Year 1, and at the end of Years 3 and 5 of their medical training. The number of students completing this instrument dropped by almost half over the course of the five years, and 'little improvement' was found as they progressed through the curriculum in terms of proposed behaviour in response to a whistleblowing scenario (Goldie *et al.* 2003, p.368). No improvement was observed on the quality of students' justifications on whether to whistleblow – unsurprising, perhaps, as the findings suggested students came into training with *negative* views of whistleblowing, a not uncommon reaction to the fate of the whistleblower in medicine. *Not* whistleblowing was associated with deference to the decisions of senior doctors (who had not blown the whistle) and awareness of the *realpolitik* of medicine and its pecking orders: if junior doctors cross paths with senior doctors they may well jeopardize their chances of getting a decent reference and blight their own career prospects. Fear of a professional backlash, of the old boys' (*sic*) network kept student doctors quiet.

As they progressed through the curriculum, the justification of these student doctors for their inaction was the 'if it's written down' rationale (possibly a close cousin to the old chestnut 'I was just obeying orders'). What *was* written down superseded what might later have been said in conversation but was *not* written down. Many students failed to recognize the ethical issues in the vignette, and instead just analysed the scenario in terms of autonomy, with little consideration of legal issues or ethical principles. They were more profoundly affected by role models than by the content of coursework (Goldie *et al.* 2003). This suggests that reflective modelling and discussion with high status colleagues might provide a way to get medical students, or others, to criticize colleagues constructively in a spirit of collegiality, rather than in non-constructive moaning or, worse, silent acquiescence in poor practice.

Hence how people *really* function and behave in the challenging worlds of health and social care is complex, conflicted, confusing and anything but the neat, linear decision-making checklist or decision tree of management training. The crude reality is that there are no consequences for trainees in the classroom. They are not staring out real world pressures such as intense scrutiny of a hostile media, lack of time and budget, punitive political or managerial imperatives that are anything but ethical in their impacts. It is not that training on ethics is wrong or out-of-place, but simply that it is sealed off from the reality that those working in health and social care services typically confront. At its most instrumental, ethics training provides cover for the organization – box ticked, people trained. But it is in the day-to-day events that the real challenge of taking and making ethical decision, of behaving morally and justly, are learned.

By definition, overcoming self-deception is a tough call for the individual. In groups, with support and validation from others, there are others around to hold up the mirror if the person cares to look in it, and reflect back self-deceiving actions and judgements. Critical questioning of behaviours and actions in workplaces that walk that talk, and in cultures that constantly question what is done and how, provide some challenge to the negative impacts of self-deception (Tenbrunsel and Messick 2004). To act ethically needs others on the same path, heading in the same direction.

THE EVIL THAT IS DONE

When she was covering the trial of Albert Eichmann, the Nazi who facilitated and organized the logistics of mass deportation and annihilation of Jews, gypsies, gay and disabled people in World War II, Arendt (1963) used the phrase 'banality of evil' to describe Eichmann's lack of remorse or any contrition about the enormity of his crimes. Eichmann insisted he had no authority in the Nazi hierarchy; that he had only been following orders as he had sworn an oath of loyalty. He admitted organizing transport to death camps but denied any responsibility for the consequences, which was the organized mass destruction of millions of people whom the Nazis hated (Cesarani 2005). He used what Arendt (2003) later came to call the cog-in-a-wheel defence: he claimed he was just one part of the Nazis' rational administration to death of those it wished to exterminate.

The 'cogism' defence has a long track record. Highly-paid news executives working for Rupert Murdoch's News Corporation who gave evidence to the Leveson Inquiry on press freedom in the UK in 2011–2012 always claimed not to know that phone hacking was a viral rot in its news-gathering media outlets (Davies 2014). Less powerful jobbing journalists, as well as their more highly paid colleagues on the company payroll, claimed that if they hadn't hacked phones, others would have. But those choosing the cogism defence – the 'if I hadn't done it, plenty more would' – are seldom, if ever, asked why they chose to be a cog and, having made that choice, went on exercising it.

The managerial metamyth of technical rationality (Ingersoll and Adams 1992), elevated to its grotesque extreme by the Nazis, is the enveloping belief that work processes should be rationalized, that efficiency is paramount, and that ends triumph over means. Technical rationality breeds standardized, chopped-up work processes. Standards influence people's judgements and how they perceive and view a situation, and fade morality from its ethical dimensions. Meeting standards and hitting targets can take on a life of their own (Ash 2014a).

In their development of the concept of 'administrative evil', Adams and Balfour (1998) identified the potential for gross harm to become embedded in those chopped-up, technocratic administrative processes. These mask the harmful outcomes this mindless pursuit of administrative efficiency, at any cost, seamlessly generates. 'Administrative evil' is doing things right by the book, even when they result in gross harm. It is the antithesis of doing the right thing. Doing one's own job brilliantly, but oblivious to its contribution to egregiously bad outcomes, is administrative evil. It leads people (those otherwise unremarkable folk discussed earlier) to delude themselves (self-deception again) into thinking that what they do is really not so bad. Within the structure of modern, complex organizations, individual responsibility is diffused, and different specialisms and departments compartmentalize tasks to get the work done, day on day. Administrative evil gets to be its most dangerous when, unnoticed (its distinguishing feature), an organization, or part of an organization falls prey to it. Failures in health and social care, such as those perpetrated by Mid Staffordshire NHS Foundation Trust, or Winterbourne View, or Rotherham Metropolitan Borough Council, all exhibited the blindness to consequence of diffusing overall responsibility for patient safety and safeguarding across a number of regulators, bodies and boards of one sort or another. Whistleblowers often find themselves as the 'voices off' in this grim pantomime, shouting, 'It's behind you!'

Humphrey (2015, p.41), in her call to face up to evil consequences, argued that two forms of societal evil were the 'crucible in which administrative evil foments'. One was cultural and ideological evil; the other structural and systemic evil. Humphrey noted the inherent vanity and self-satisfaction to be found in the uncritical acceptance and hot pursuit of latest fads and fancies of organizational and business life by leaders and politicians. She called for a deeper, critical reflection of the impacts of political and managerial *zeitgeists* (public expenditure-slashing, austerity, the privatization of public goods such as health and social care, are but some). It is the unspoken motives of governments and employers that require our critical interrogation, as it is in these that the bases of so many unintended impacts of administrative evil emanate (Humphrey 2015).

Bauman argued that the Holocaust provided a means to understand how formal and ethically blind the bureaucratic pursuit of efficiency can be: 'At no point of its long and tortuous execution did the Holocaust come in conflict with the principles of rationality' (Bauman 1989, p.17). Sociology, too, with its rational scientific bent, fell in with the moral silence of science. Milgram's work on obedience, discussed in the previous chapter, has been excoriated by the scientific community for its findings, illustrating 'the reality of the allegedly value-free search for knowledge and disinterested motives of scientific curiosity' (Bauman 1989, p.152). Yet the real, deep learning from Milgram's obedience studies was that cruelty wasn't done by evil monsters but by ordinary, otherwise decent, and apparently socially adjusted people. This cruelty does not correlate with personality or psychometric tests and profiles, but strongly with the relationships of authority, dominance and subordination between people. Ask the person in the street their views and they will express abhorrence at the dehumanization of innocent adults and children;

yet they may do things with precisely these impacts when ordered to by an authority. Behaviour that is abhorrent in an individual who is acting on his or her own may be performed without demur when carried out under orders.

Inside bureaucratic systems of authority the language of morality gets a new twist, with loyalty, duty, discipline pre-eminent in the dominant/subordinate relationships of authority and subordination. The subordinate feels shame or pride in their work in line with how the dominant authority judges them. It is not the goodness or badness of actions but the compliance with instruction and direction that counts: 'Bureaucracy's double feat is the moralization of technology, coupled with the denial of the moral significance of non-technical issues' (Bauman 1989, p.160).

One of Milgram's obedience experiments involved the actors in authority roles openly arguing with each other, in front of the volunteer who was being asked to administer the electric shocks they were told were real (Bauman 1989). When they heard this arguing, more volunteers stopped administering (the fake) electric shocks at an earlier point – as if they had found chinks in the armour of those giving orders, and thus could behave more humanely. It is the total, monopolistic nature of authority that influences a person to act against their own conscience and espoused value system. For Bauman (1989), the Milgram experiments showed that pluralism, different points of view, and more than one way of doing something, provided better preventive protection against the propensity of morally normal people to do abnormally immoral acts. Cruelty correlates more with certain patterns of social interaction (such as command and control), than with individual personality traits of otherwise unremarkable people. In this way cruelty, or, at a less extreme end, turning a blind eye to poor practice, originates in social interaction and in relationships of power, control and subordination, and not in personality characteristics. Rationality, obeying orders, doing as one is told in the authority relationships of bureaucracies and large organizations, mostly trumps behaving in ethical ways. Deviating from this becomes the whistleblower's lot, or fate.

ORGANIZATIONAL BLIND SPOTS

If insanity is doing the same wrong thing over and over again and expecting different results, then blind spots – not seeing or looking away – are protective shields from the disconnect of doing something over and over again, yet knowing it doesn't work. In organizations, these blind spots are present when leaders, managers and employees cannot acknowledge strategies that do not work. By failing to do this, they 'sustain an illusory possibility of success' (Fotaki and Hyde 2015, p.441), committing to failing strategies, the impact of which on those far beyond the organization is huge, whether on patients, employees, the general public. It is often the whistleblower who says things are not what they seem: the emperor is without clothes.

Fotaki and Hyde (2015) had two broad explanations for this paradox: first, the psychological tendency of individuals to believe they are objective and balanced in their subjective perceptions of people and things (perception bias); and second, our psychological difficulty in accepting previous losses, or mistakes, or bad calls of one sort or another. As with the gambler who goes on playing when the chips are down, there is a psychological tendency to keep going, thinking luck will turn.

Fotaki and Hyde (2015) called these social and psychological defences against the anxiety of failure and failing 'organizational blind spots'. Organizational blind spots describe the organization's staying committed to something unworkable. These blind spots are formed when unrealistic policies are formed in response to unconscious social demands – for example, that health systems should prevent disease and death. Blind spots are fuelled by psychological defence mechanisms that maintain the commitment to failing strategies, such as splitting (where a person unconsciously splits off unpleasant realizations from an idealized positive), blaming others and idealizing. These social defences are reinforced in the wider social and policy environment, where people and groups reproduce them. Blind spots aren't denial in itself, but its institutionalization through the routines, ritual and storytelling of workplace life. In not acknowledging organizational failings, the feelings attached to them are split off and projected onto someone or someplace else. Responsibility and blame are placed elsewhere, allowing the organization to continue its pursuit of the unworkable. When reality dawns, more blame may be heaped on the outsiders or insiders who did not buy into the narrative.

Fotaki and Hyde (2015) were considering psychosocial dimensions of organizational blind spots and failure within the social, structural, policy and political backdrop that frames them. The dangerous paradox is, of course, that, by definition, policy makers and politicians do not recognize the blind spots in the projects, plans and policies that they promote, any more than they recognize self-deception (Heffernan 2011). A wilful turning away and reluctance to acknowledge blind spots ensures their survival and proliferation. Understanding and expecting blind spots to be present, and tackling the resistance and ignorance that may reinforce them – for example, by paying attention to contrary voices, counter-arguments, and to whistleblowers – are one means to mitigate the damage blind spots inflict on people and work.

HEALTH AND SOCIAL CARE DISASTERS

Healthcare disasters, such as the failures of healthcare of Mid Staffordshire NHS Foundation Trust in England between 2005 and 2009, are inevitably followed by inquiries and investigations that set out the signs, signals, raised concerns, that were missed, misunderstood or mismanaged by professionals, leaders and managers paid to monitor the safety and quality of care (Francis Report 2013a, b, c; Mid Staffordshire NHS Foundation Trust Inquiry 2010). If it is the case that this failure to pay attention was not intended to cause the harm and suffering that occurred, it follows that those responsible for leading, improving and regulating patient safety need to be a bit more alert to the need to identify, interpret and act on the early warnings and weak signals of emerging risks, before those risks result in a disastrous failure of care. Macrae (2014a) argued that these challenges are organizational and cultural; they pivot on what information is routinely noticed, communicated and attended to within and between healthcare organizations and, most critically, what is assumed and ignored.

Observing that 'disasters are essentially organised events', Macrae (2014a, p.441) said they follow systematic and prolonged neglect of warning signs and signals of danger, creating 'deep pockets of organisational ignorance, organisational silence and organisational blindness'. When signals of risk are not noticed, or are misunderstood, then the safeguards and defences against those risks are weakened, assuming they existed in the first place.

Macrae's (2014b) work on 'close calls' in aircraft safety provides a powerful crossover into health and social care. *Contra* the eye-wateringly expensive, inevitably delayed, after-the-event inquiries of health and social care when things have gone wrong, airline flight safety investigators continually scrutinize flight data. They observe both the mundane and the extreme. This work requires expertise that is both broad and deep; it needs creative thinking alongside the capacities to be suspicious, curious and endlessly probing. In flight safety, like health or social care, early warning signs are often humdrum, minor and easy to miss in the absence of the vigilance that is supported and expected in the organizational culture. A lack of general cleanliness, rough ways of speaking to patients and users of health or social care services, poor hygiene practices, are all signs of slippage which, left unchecked, can quickly deteriorate into major, life-threatening incidents, such as patient death from a hospital-acquired infection. Organizational disasters incubate over long periods of time: they don't spontaneously combust as bizarre or unfathomable acts. It is precisely those events, occurrences and circumstances that do not sit with conventional wisdom, those shorthand ways of doing things, the familiar group norms and pressures that don't get noticed or attended to. Disasters develop, in other words, through sustained and systemic failures of interpretation and attention (Macrae 2014a).

Some of these missed, miscommunicated or misinterpreted signals of risk are closed professional cultures that exclude those voices off saying the emperor is without clothes. Nurses, doctors, social workers and managers on the ground, as it were, are more likely than not to know where the problems are and where the risks are, and to have concerns of varying degrees of severity, in relation to patient safety and care quality. The 2013 Francis Report on Mid Staffordshire NHS Foundation Trust recounted many of the fears of doctors who knew of problems of care but kept quiet, because to raise these would be (they believed) career suicide, or because they feared they would be regarded as complicit (guilt by association) in what was going on. It seemed safer to walk on by, rather than be called upon to justify, defend and explain failures they may have witnessed, and so face blame by complicity.

Health and social care staff are well used to working in organizations and systems that are far from some idealized confection of compassionate care. There is never enough time; equipment and resources may be old; demand often exceeds capacity. Muddling through, getting by, putting up with, become survival strategies to deliver the service. Superimpose onto this a proliferation of overlapping regulatory bodies, the political football that is free-at-the-point-of-delivery national healthcare in the UK, and then, as happened in Mid Staffordshire NHS Foundation Trust, conditions ripen to incubate disasters. If risks and warning signs are not attended to and recognized for what they are, the rot can set in.

Macrae (2014a) said that in healthcare this slow incubation provides the opportunity to take action before disaster occurs – but only if attention and resources are mobilized. For this to happen requires, first, that there is a hunger – an overwhelming desire – to spot problems and early warning signs *throughout* the organization (not just at the frontline, service delivery end); second, that there are effective monitoring systems to pick these up; and third – critically – that there are the will and capacity to put right, with intelligence and commitment, the systemic problems that underlie disasters.

The events and problems that the 2013 Francis Report identified in Mid Staffordshire NHS Foundation Trust provided a masterclass in what and how disasters occur. Complaints and patient safety were mishandled, instead of being regarded as providing valid, valuable information for anyone who was alert, vigilant, and paying attention to what was going on. Whistleblowers were discouraged; those raising concerns were blamed, bullied or threatened. One of the Francis Report's recommendations was that reporting and information collection needed overhaul. Except that the Mid Staffordshire NHS Foundation Trust had overloads of information. In a three-month period between January and March 2007, the Trust had a patient safety incident concerning staffing levels *every day*. Staff, far from keeping quiet, were raising these; data were collected *ad nauseam*. But when data aren't interrogated with expertise, competence and a detached curiosity, when pieces of information are used to bolster up the shop window façade for a regulator, rather than to inform intelligent, thoughtful leadership and management, they become little more than costly, useless bric-à-brac. They cease to be used, useful, or usable. When daily patient safety incidents are ignored, passed on and then passed over, when the messenger is blamed for the message, there is a problem, and it is systemic, and it is one for those who did not pay attention to the reports they were given.

SYSTEMATIC ATTENTION DEFICIT DISORDER

This problem might be understood as a systemic attention deficit disorder. As Macrae (2014a) commented, improving the capture, analysis and presentation of information on safety and quality cannot be anything other than important, in the same way as being clear of the mandate (as if it were not already so) that governance and regulatory infrastructures have to *interpret* and *use* the information they have. It is their job. It is what they are paid to do. It cannot be otherwise. But problems lie at deeper, systemic levels, where social and cognitive processes and systems interpret – make sense of – the information. Mid Staffordshire NHS Foundation Trust used information to support their bid to achieve foundation trust status, to construct a false narrative of safety and quality that discounted the counter-factuals presented by those raising concerns. In order to monitor and ensure quality and safety, the systems, processes and people who operate and work in them have to pay attention, with intention, to data that challenge, disconfirm and question those expedient assumptions and convenient wisdoms. As in the matter of airline safety, assumptions and beliefs about safety and quality of health and social care have to be explicit – and continually challenged – within those organizations and their regulators. Early warning signs from staff, disconfirming data and information, need attention and amplification. Paying attention and acknowledging ignorance are the friends, not foes, of the governance and regulator structures (Macrae 2014a).

Getting wise and tackling this systematic attention deficit disorder means looking for and paying attention to early warning signs in health and social care systems. It means creating organizational cultures that reward, value and expect employees to speak out about poor care. It is not some complex and esoteric practice that lies outside what happens now in health and social care systems. It doesn't cost money. One of the understandable complaints of those criticized in the inevitable inquiries and re-inspections that follow disasters in health and social care, is that people knew what was going on, and that they tried to get something done to put it right. But this intelligence becomes mushed-up with prettily presented graphs and bar charts whose aim is to convince others of the health of the organization (even when information embedded in them tells an entirely different story). Warning signs don't appear in neat red packages with 'danger' stencilled down the side. Warning signs have to be constructed as such to get attention, and have to be related to pre-existing concerns about potential failures and future harm. *Expecting* problems, *looking* for failure, stands more of chance of producing what Macrae (2014a) called the 'right kind of fear' – fear that is motivated by the pursuit of quality and safety, not the paralysing dread of trial by public opprobrium. Mobilizing staff, managers and leaders to be clear about what should be avoided helps detection and rectification of the what-is-to-be-avoided. If staffing levels are constantly too low, if people consistently receive fewer or worse services than they need, if equipment is regularly not available, then these are warning signs that should galvanize attention and prompt action.

What happened in Mid Staffordshire NHS Foundation Trust, in Winterbourne View care home and Rotherham Metropolitan Borough Council in England, comes out of system-wide meltdowns, as well as individual and human misdoings that span health and social care systems, from regulators, commissioners, providers, professionals, politicians and the rest. Each plays its part in the success, and the appalling failures, that may occur. After any airline accident or serious incident, the matter is routinely investigated by independent airline safety specialists. Not lawyers, not members of the establishment, not worthy public figures, but people who know their business, who aren't attached to the airline or its management, and whose investigation takes in the system and infrastructure surrounding the problem (Macrae 2014b). The airline industry is fiercely competitive and commercial. Its bottom lines take an immediate hit when disasters occur and lives are lost. In health and social care, the stakes are equally high; and it is the whistleblower who may provide the early warning of problems that, if not resolved, may cost lives.

CHAPTER 6

HOW NOT TO ENCOURAGE WHISTLEBLOWING

The organizational and political reaction to the whistleblower can be, as we have seen, conflicted. Mournful regret that people did not step forward sooner (some employees probably did, but were silenced or simply not heard), or excoriation of frontline staff (seldom those employed to lead the service) deemed responsible for the perpetration of serious harm and wrongdoing, are now stock-in-trade responses of politicians and national leaders following public exposure of a scandal in health and social care. The reasons why people do not speak out, any appreciation of the significance of power, authority and obedience in the workplace, and of the social need for people to fit in and conform to the organizational culture in which they find themselves, are seldom, if ever, the focus of thoughtful, considered reflection following a disaster.

Some set piece solutions are often offered up to deal with the challenge that whistleblowing poses to organizations that really don't want their dirty washing to see light of day. These include the sticks and carrots of financially monetizing whistleblowing, and of laying a contractual or regulatory duty on employees to speak out. The former throws money at the problem without being clear about what exactly the problem is. The latter is an exquisite Catch 22: the individual is damned both if they do, and if they don't, speak out. It is inevitable, of course, that various solutions are put forward in the aftermath of a scandal or disaster in health or social care. It is *not* inevitable that the 'solutions' adopted are devoid of evidence that they may do anything other than further undermine trust in the workplace. Lewis (2011) was right to say that the development of whistleblowing law and policy needs a rethink of what counts as trust and loyalty in the workplace, and the same goes for policy reactions to scandals.

This chapter discusses the periodically popular 'cash for whistleblowing' and 'duty to whistleblow' responses to the 'this must never happen again' post-disaster pieties so often proffered by politicians and organizational leaders. This discussion notes that neither of these proposals considers, still less provides, a 'solution' (*sic*) to the deeper organizational dynamics that are turning the blind eye, or the deaf ear, to problems of care, including its resourcing. The potential impacts of these two proposals on 'trust' that employees and the general public have in these organizations remain unexamined. Putting some cash in a whistleblowing kitty, or holding the individual responsible for speaking out, fails to grasp the impacts of the social dynamics at work in organizations. The chapter argues that creating a mandatory 'duty to whistleblow' and increased regulation following a scandal, mistakenly conflate public and employee trust in health and social care services with this 'confidence apparatus', and that trust in such apparatus is misplaced.

CASH FOR WHISTLEBLOWING

When things go wrong in health and social care, and whether or not that problem has been processed through whistleblowing legislation, the wrongdoing is seldom something that people working near to the problem were unaware of. As we have seen, staff in the Mid Staffordshire NHS Foundation Trust were raising concerns about patient care for years before Robert Francis QC was asked to carry out his public inquiry into what went wrong (Francis 2013a).

Given the long-lasting career- and livelihood-destroying experiences of many whistleblowers, to contemplate the possibility of rewarding them – financially – for raising the concerns they did, seems odd. It is not a proposal that most of those with experience of whistleblowing (from either side of the disclosure fence, so to speak), or those working in organizations who advise and support whistleblowers, favour. PCaW, the UK whistleblowing charity, found little support among those who gave evidence to its Whistleblowing Commission for financially rewarding someone for speaking out about wrongdoing (PCaW 2013). The same finding came out of the 2014 survey of NHS workers carried out as part of Robert Francis's *Freedom to Speak Up* review; this found NHS staff had no appetite for systems that financially rewarded whistleblowers for speaking out (Lewis, D'Angelo and Clarke 2015).

Throwing cash around in this way does not sit easily with the typical way of doing the business of health and social care in the UK, at least in the non-profit and public sectors. It is a solution that fundamentally fails to grasp the problem. The failures of health and social care discussed in this book, such as Mid Staffordshire NHS Foundation Trust, Winterbourne View, Rotherham Metropolitan Borough Council, were systemic, organizational and cultural. They occurred in organizational cultures that reinforced the dysfunctional inversion of care that these places came to represent. Sure, organizations can put cash in the hand of the person who speaks out, but first they have to ask why it is that those who have spoken out in the past have come to such a sticky end. Organizations have to ask of themselves why signs and signals of poor practice are not picked up routinely and regularly; or if they are, why they are ignored; and why day-to-day discourse of the team, department and its management is not focused on spotting and rectifying these matters in the first place.

It is not too great a stretch of the imagination to see how financially rewarding the whistleblower is likely to backfire on them. The organization that considers using money in this way may well be one where the whistleblower finds that others accuse them of 'only doing it for the money'. Anyone else contemplating raising concerns about practice is unlikely to be encouraged by this. Using cash to tackle the problems of organizational silence, of the blind eye and deaf ear of workplace life, can end up with false, or delayed, reporting of wrongdoing. And if a case goes before the courts, the first line of attack, the *ad hominem* demolition of the character and motives of the whistleblower by the defence barrister, is likely to be, 'You did it for the money didn't you?'

A DUTY TO REPORT

If not financial rewards to entice whistleblowing, then laying a duty – a mandatory obligation – on an employee to speak out is another proposal put forward post-disaster. As it is, regulated health and social care employees have a duty to report poor care and, as noted earlier, a duty of candour was laid on health employees in England in 2015. Whilst it is ostensibly, and absolutely, appropriate that regulated, responsible professionals speak up when standards slip, a duty to report places the employee in another double bind. They are held responsible for their moral behaviour, yet they lack moral autonomy, as their employing organization creates, oversees and polices the systems and processes employees are required to follow. People do not work in a vacuum; their autonomy is mediated and managed through professional duties, incentives, rewards, colleague and manager support, workplace and peer group norms. 'Moral agency' isn't immaculate conception; it is socially formed, socially situated and socially reinforced within the organizational cultures of the workplace. If employees are be regarded as either responsible or liable for wrongdoing, then the significant influence of the situation and context in which they work needs to hold a mirror responsibility.

The 'at first sight' attraction of responses to wrongdoing, paying the whistleblower, making people whistleblow, sits on some deeper contradictions. Tsahuridu and Vandekerckhove (2008) identified two of these. In the first, whistleblowing legislation and policies are regarded as facilitating individual responsibility and moral autonomy at work. In the second, this same statutory infrastructure protects the organization by controlling employees and making *them* liable for upholding ethics in the workplace. To unravel this conundrum, Tsahuridu and Vandekerckhove drew on Bauman's (1993) concept of 'ethical distance' to examine the impact of whistleblowing policies on moral autonomy. 'Ethical distance' is the distance between the person as a moral agent, and the wrongdoing or the harmful circumstances. Tsahuridu and Vandekerckhove argued that while whistleblowing policies find justification as an organizational device to enhance the moral autonomy of people at work, implementing these policies can turn that responsibility into a *liability* for the employee.

INDIVIDUAL AUTONOMY, INDIVIDUAL LIABILITY

The metamorphosis that transforms autonomy into liability presents another double bind for the employee, as set out by Tsahuridu and Vandekerckhove (2008). Organizational whistleblowing policies lay down procedures to be followed when raising concerns. These reinforce the notion of ethical distance between people in organizations and organizational outcomes, but in what Tsahuridu and Vandekerckhove said were two contradictory ways. First, whistleblowing policies and procedures can increase the ethical distance between the person speaking out and the wrongdoing: by raising their concerns under these policies the whistleblower seeks to be distanced from the wrongdoing. But, second, and paradoxically, in providing a means for employees to speak out about concerns, whistleblowing policies may decrease ethical distance in the organization, everyone who knows about potential wrongdoing then shares responsibility for doing something about it. The conceptual conundrum is this: a right to whistleblow increases ethical distance; a duty to whistleblow decreases ethical distance.

This is more than mere semantics. Whistleblowing policies – generally considered to be morally acceptable – set out the processes by which employees can raise concerns, and be afforded some protection against detriment when they do. But if those policies make employees responsible for voicing concerns they are, in fact, laying a duty on employees to disclose potential wrongdoing. Morally, the question becomes whether, and how, employees can be held responsible for organizational wrongdoing, over which they have no control. Gifting employees with responsibility for whistleblowing may thus become a liability, albeit one dressed up as autonomy. In these circumstances, if they do not speak out (and there are many good reasons why they may not, whistleblowing policy or not), the employee is held to account. When this happens, as Tsahuridu and Vandekerckhove (2008, p.115) noted, whistleblowing policies become 'another tool in the hands of organisations to control employee behaviour: a reduction in autonomy. The policies can also offer protection to the organisation by shifting responsibility of organisational behaviour to individual members'.

PROBLEMS OF A 'DUTY TO WHISTLEBLOW'

Employees and professionals held to account through their professional codes of conduct or through contractual obligations to their employer may, of course, work in organizations that do not have whistleblowing policies and procedures that provide effective protection for the person raising concerns. The obligations all seem tilted one way, and that is away from the employer. As Bouville (2008, p.585) observed: 'Codes that make whistle-blowing mandatory are like generals that send soldiers to be killed: the one giving the order does not suffer any adverse consequences. Telling others to sacrifice themselves is no sacrifice.' The Whistleblowing Commission of PCaW (2013), referred to earlier, considered whether a code of practice should make it mandatory for workers to blow the whistle about poor or corrupt practice. The Commission concluded that whilst it is commonplace for duties to report malpractice or wrongdoing to be attached to certain professions (for example, doctors, nurses, lawyers, accountants), an overarching 'duty to blow the whistle' may cause more problems than it solves. It may encourage over-reporting, countenance scapegoating, or lead to organizations hunting down those who did not speak up, rather than addressing the root problem of wrongdoing, or the overall effectiveness of the organization's whistleblowing arrangements.

Other difficulties arise when a duty to report is imposed on employees. Lewis (2010) wondered if action would be taken against an employee who tried to comply with this duty, but lacked sufficient evidence to make a full disclosure. Or would it be the case that those who did not report wrongdoing, because they did not regard it as such, would be sanctioned or disciplined? The impact of sanctions and duties to report, in a workplace climate and culture where organizational silence, turning a blind eye and fitting in with one's colleagues, come what may, all operate under the radar of procedures, codes and duties, is hard to call. Sanctioning systems impact on cooperative behaviour and the teamwork that is vital to the delivery of health and social care. Sanctions affect the type of decision people perceive they are making: taking action becomes an organizational requirement (box ticked), and not an ethical decision about the quality of care provided (Tenbrunsel and Messick 1999).

In any case, for any organization the challenge is how to create systems that achieve compliance. Monitoring behaviour, surveillance, reward and punishment are the usual *modi operandi*. While a lot of time and huge amounts of money are involved in running them, these systems probably do not function as well as the claims made for them would suggest. It is typically social reinforcement that powerfully conditions people. Weak sanctions intended to increase cooperation may actually reduce it, as they lack credibility. Strong sanctions may increase cooperation, but the basis for this cooperation is different: it is cooperation for business rather than ethical reasons – doing things right rather than doing the right thing (Tenbrunsel and Messick 1999). It is hardly a surprise that the evidence on the effectiveness of formal codes to reduce wrongdoing is mixed (Tenbrunsel, Smith-Crowe and Umphress 2003). Compliance is not a synonym for ethical action.

Dissonance, and the jarring of personal commitment to ethical right action, can be the upshot when rules and regulations obscure the essentially human dimensions of health and social care (Bauman 2000). Rules and regulations obfuscate the moral impetus and drive that underlie this work in health and social care. Codes, duties and responsibilities all, very rationally, allow for sanctions to be levied against those who do not comply. But rationality is not morality. Morality cannot be operationalized, measured and standardized in the way of rationality and rules: 'morality is endemically and irredeemably non-rational – in the sense of not being calculable, hence not being presentable as following impersonal rules' (Bauman 1993, p.60). Ambiguity and uncertainty occupy the terrain of the ethical world, and certainly the reality of daily work and decisions work in health and social care services (Bauman 2000). It is in that ambiguity and uncertainty that the potential for moral action is located, not in rules, duties and regulations. They are the means but not the end. As Smith (2011, p.15) had it, 'Merely following rules/procedures gets us off the hook of proper moral endeavour. Morality needs to be grounded and demonstrated within relationships and through moral comportment within these.' Rules are certainly necessary, but they are not sufficient to deliver ethical care in the workplace.

COMPLIANCE, CONFIDENCE AND CODES

Other tricky issues arise with the 'compliance and the codes' spirit of the times in health and social care. The codes of professional practice with which registered health and social care practitioners comply are not unproblematic. For Vandekerckhove (2014) these codes were both reactive (to something that happened in the past), and defensive (in place to provide organizational protection). In their reactive mode, codes originate from a past problem: something that has occurred. As a defence, they are adopted because other organizations have them and, as they are a statutory requirement, any sanctions on an organization having these in place are likely to be less severe than if they were not in place. Codes exist to protect the organization from sanction, not to promote right action in its work. Reactivity and defensiveness are hardly positive bases for bedding integrity into the moral functioning of an organization: compliance-based codes and obligations are the lowest common denominator of ethical organizational functioning. As Vandekerckhove (2012) observed, what health and social care needs is not managers and employees solely of the code-compliance persuasion, but managers and employees who behave and act ethically – in other words, with integrity.

TRUSTING THE CONFIDENCE APPARATUS

The bureaucratic apparatus of regulation, standards, compliance, clinical and organizational governance structures is intended to give citizens trust in health and social care systems. The unaddressed problem with all this, aside from the bizarre promise to do more of the same that did not prevent a given disaster occurring any more than it did a previous one, is the conflation of rebuilding trust with tightening standards and regulation. Public trust and confidence in public institutions and political classes are based on rather more than codes of practice, and standards of this or that. Trust is a complex, affective, nuanced, sensed and felt, social and personal phenomenon that takes many forms. Dusty, tired organizational straplines and last year's (or last decade's) posters proclaiming 'What you can expect from us' are as near to trust-building as are repetitive proclamations of sorry-saying and lesson-learning after disasters. These empty promises miss the point. Trust is created in real time, in real life, in the interplay of interactions and relationships between people and social systems (Fotaki 2014).

The proliferation of standards, regulation and inspection of health and social care services in the UK since the 1990s has conflated these with public confidence and trust. This apparatus stands between the whistleblower and the citizen at risk of suffering harm or worse. It consumes itself. Collecting data to show, one way or another, that targets have been met, becomes the end, rather than the practice or process of health and social care delivery. Increased bureaucratization and surveillance claim to demonstrate effectiveness, to pick out the best and worst. They are supposed to provide citizens with the means to *trust* sectors and services. Trust is certainly needed when the elements of social interaction lack certainty, but it is not located in a cost–benefit, in/out checklist of probabilities in situations of uncertainty generated by some Orwellian Ministry of Trust. Trusting a doctor, social worker, care worker, nurse, paramedic (rather than simply submitting to their ministrations) involves risk and some personal judgement about personal attributes.

In differentiating between trust and confidence, Harrison and Smith (2004) characterized *trust* as relationships between people, and *confidence* as found in the relationships between people and systems. The more these systems and their experts are depended upon, the less uncertainty arises, and the less trust is relied upon. Trust involves vulnerability – not knowing with complete certainty that x will follow y. Trust hinges on free will and discretion: in trusting something of the self to others we have to credit them with being able and willing to make judgements about how to care for us.

In this way of looking at trust in health and social care, there thus arises a clear relationship between trust and morality. Abstract systems cannot act or manifest moral agency; morality exists outside abstract systems. Trust *is* moral, and risk is present along with vulnerability, individual agency, discretion and an absence of the instrumental trappings of regulation. Trust becomes even more significant when action cannot effectively be governed by regulation, or relied on with confidence (Harrison and Smith 2004).

This is obviously critical in health and social care. If *trust* is lost, or replaced, as the means by which health and care are provided to citizens, a number of negative unintended consequences arise. First, transaction costs explode, as a costly legal and regulatory apparatus springs to life to provide a substitute for trust. When we replace trust, human responsiveness and kindness with the apparatus of confidence, the risks and costs of litigation rise. Second, the confidence apparatus provides misplaced certainty – the fig leaf response. Responding to the complexity and unpredictability of human endeavour and mishap is nothing if not an exercise in being present with uncertainty. The focus – the point – of the confidence apparatus are calculable bottom-line possibilities, resulting in misplaced expectation that that apparatus *itself* is something in which public trust can be placed. The inevitable conflict between satisfying auditors and dealing with uncertainty can result in the practitioner doing the defensible – that which can be justified, explained and defended – in precedence to what may be right in all the circumstances. Third, abstract systems and instrumental reason put means before ends. Generating and controlling knowledge and power hasn't much interest in moral ends. Behaving in a moral way that generates trust becomes extrinsic to the endeavour, not the measured means to deliver the desirable end (Giddens 1990; Harrison and Smith 2004).

This confidence apparatus is shrouded in a lot of *faux* moral window dressing. Grand statements about vision, social responsibility, putting citizens first, are spray-painted onto rules, as if to cover the cracks. Rules alone cannot respond to the adult or child who is raped, harmed or maltreated, to the person living in constant life-limiting pain, or the patient near to death. The affective human traits needed in professionals and anyone supporting the adult or child through this process – all well beyond the operational scope of the outputs of the confidence apparatus industry – are likely to include compassion, kindness, tact, competence, honesty, truthfulness. Engaging with vulnerable citizens, adults or children at these times requires giving them full attention. This is a moral matter, not one for the governance checklist, the mandatory, audited completion of which professionals are judged accountable for (rather than carrying accountability for moral action). This is not to suggest soft, affective matters are to be elevated over technical competence, knowledge and demonstrable performance; but rather both are needed to deliver health and care services that are both moral and competent.

PREVENTION IS BETTER THAN CURE

Organizations probably get the trust, and the respect, they deserve. Many organizational managers who receive internal reports of wrongdoing (for example, HR; middle managers) think a large proportion of complaints have no merit, even when this is not the case (Miceli and Near 2005). If organizational leadership and human resources functions are distrustful, then disclosure of wrongdoing by an employee will be clouded in self-questioning about whether it is worth the detriment that the worker may find themselves subject to, whatever the policies of cash for whistleblowing or duties to report may have to say.

Neither the carrot of cash incentives to whistleblow, nor the stick of the duty to report, really comprehend the influence of the organizational culture, and cultures, on trust in the workplace, and on the behaviour and actions of those who work in it. Most employees who observe wrongdoing in organizations do not report it to someone who can take corrective action. They will be more likely to do so when they work in an organizational culture they experience as reasonable and fair – one they can trust. In a setting like this, where managers observably and demonstrably take action to stop poor practice and right wrongdoing, employees feel more supported and regard the organization as more just. This is win–win: organizations that are experienced as fair and supportive by those who work in them, are rewarded with greater employee commitment, trust and engagement in service improvement, and in speaking out about its failures (Miceli *et al.* 2012). They are unlikely to have much use for cash for whistleblowing policies.

Where organizational wrongdoing is not normalized or institutionalized, a high employee commitment to the organization and its values is more likely to encourage whistleblowing, because the observed wrongdoing is at odds with things as usual. Employees with a low identification with the organization are less likely to whistleblow; whereas those who identify with it, and have longer tenure (and thus potentially more confidence in their judgement) are more likely to be successful in getting others on side to draw attention to and stop wrongdoing (Miceli, Near and Dworkin 2008). An organization whose culture rewards and reinforces its managers to behave ethically is likely to be one where problems are attended to earlier, before they become disasters. Those managers can do a number of things to embed trust and to encourage moral agency in the workforce. They can behave as moral agents themselves; and they can expect their peers, bosses and subordinates to do likewise. They can create and police tough anti-retaliation policies to protect the whistleblower from retaliation, and to sanction those who attempt it. They can orient employees to what the organization considers to be wrong; beat the drum to the need to raise concerns; and they can reinforce that behaviour when people do. When concerns are expressed, they can focus on the wrongdoing, not on the person raising it (or their sickness absence record, or their travel claim history. Any problems with those would have been picked up when they arose by the ethical manager). They will investigate fairly and fully; and take swift, corrective action when the complaint is well-founded (Miceli *et al.* 2008).

To propose an instrumental fix-it such as financially rewarding whistleblowers for speaking out is to sidestep the significance of both organizational culture in framing and shaping how people do their jobs, and of the level of trust employees and those reliant on its services have in the organization. When an organization's leaders and managers behave authentically, credibly and ethically in their dealings with employees, and with those who rely on the organizations they lead for health and social care, with the wider public, those behaviours set the bar for others. This way of acting is not the behaviour of a saint. These are not superhuman qualities. They are, rather, dependably human. These are attributes of fallibility, of curiosity, of questioning and of an overarching impulse towards the achievement of best outcomes for people using health and social care services, and against organizational cover-up of harm. What the dimensions and shape of such ethical leadership are or might be is set out in Chapter 8. Before that discussion, in considering how an ethical pulse can beat throughout health and care services and systems, the next chapter examines how an ethic of care may inform the leadership, management and delivery of ethical care.

CHAPTER 7

WHISTLEBLOWING IN ETHICAL HEALTH AND SOCIAL CARE SYSTEMS

Since the 1990s the UK has seen an upsurge of commentary and chatter talk about ethics and standards (although these are not the same thing), alongside an increase in regulation of health and social care services, including parts of their workforces that were previously unregulated. Organizational and business ethics, or 'rules or principles that define right and wrong conduct' (Davis and Frederick 1984, p.76) have become a standard feature of management and leadership education and training programmes. Often delivered by means of case studies (typically of financial misdemeanour, or a life-and-death scenario), and usually by people who are well paid, protected, safe and secure from the consequences and costs of unethical organizational practices, or of raising them, the concerned conclusions reached in these trainings will be far away from the broken marriages, impoverishment, life- and career-wrecking personal disparagement whistleblowers so often suffer.

Drawing on themes developed thus far in this book – the significance of *context* and of *social* relationships to organizational culture and whistleblowing – this chapter makes the case for ethical behaviour – right action – to manifest *throughout* the health and social care systems that patients or service users, employees, managers and leaders, as well as the whistleblower, find themselves in. The chapter's principal focus is consideration of how an ethic of care – specifically the elements of a care ethic originally put forward by Berenice Fisher and Joan Tronto, and expanded subsequently by Tronto (Fisher and Tronto 1990; Tronto 1993, 2013) might create and sustain ethically-driven health and social care service systems. It draws on and expands the ideas initially put forward by Ash (2010, 2011, 2014b, 2015). These wider health and social care systems include public policy and regulation of health and social care; the organizations and services that employ health and social care professionals and others, as well as health and social care delivered directly to citizens. If an ethic of care is to be integral, rather than a bolt-on apologia, to public policy making, then the role of government in creating a backdrop for caregiving within an ethical frame is self-evident. Listening, responding, paying attention, building frameworks of care are, ethically, integral to the job of policy making and politics. Throughout, this discussion recognizes the essentially collaborative and relational dimensions of health and social care: caring for the health and wellbeing of others is working together – throughout health and social care systems – to alleviate suffering, or at least do no more harm.

DEFINING ETHICS AND MORALITY

'Morality' does not have a standard definition in the field of behavioural ethics. Rest (1986, p.3), for example, used morality to mean a 'particular type of social value, that having to do with how humans cooperate and coordinate their activities in the service of furthering welfare, and how they adjudicate conflicts among individual interests'. Behavioural ethics as a field of study is concerned with individual behaviour that is judged or appraised within accepted moral norms of behaviour (Treviño, Weaver and Reynolds 2006). Behaviours judged unethical within this frame might include lying, stealing and cheating, as well as failing to meet a moral standard; ethical behaviours might include charitable giving or helping others without any expectation of payment or favour. To get to where ethics and the whistleblower meet, however, needs a bit more deep digging to understand the behaviours and the dynamics that exist within those social relations.

THE WHISTLEBLOWER AS ETHICAL CANARY

Miners took canaries with them into mines to provide early warning of the escape of carbon monoxide and other noxious gases. If the canary died, the miners had notice to get out of the pit fast. People working in organizations, not only the whistleblower, often hear, see and witness poor or corrupt practices that, if attended to, could provide organizations with the early warning that systems, structures and processes are not working as they should. Like the canary, the whistleblower is often the one who pays the price for alerting the organization to problems.

Those experiences and that victimization of many whistleblowers give us pause to ask how health and social care provision is to be planned and delivered to achieve the moral purposes that do no more harm, and are the alleviation of suffering and provision of care and support for sick or vulnerable people. Morality is threaded through the lives we lead, the work we do, and the care and love we give and receive, in and outside health and social care. Walker (2007, p.ix) was of the view that 'we cannot understand morality and moral belief without recognizing that moral understandings will be expressed through social ones and that social identities and roles will include moral understandings as working parts'. Developing her 'expressive collaborative model' as a template for moral inquiry, Walker (2007) suggested people learn to understand each other and express understandings in what she called 'practices of responsibility', where they accept or deflect responsibilities for different things. These practices involve making moral judgements of each other, paying attention, visiting blame, making excuses, making amends; all ways in which we express senses of responsibility. For Walker, morality was fundamentally *interpersonal* and *collaborative*: it is produced, reproduced and modified in what goes on between or among people. Morality exists in practices that show what is valued.

To act with integrity in health and social care calls up profoundly moral questions. Is integrity doing what you think is right? Or what someone else says is right? What a statutory professional code says is right? Is integrity the justification of ends over means? Personal integrity cannot exist outside a wider view of morality and moral justification. Walker (2007) regarded this as 'interpersonal', or a kind of reliable accountability and resilient dependability. Such 'reliable accountability' rests on integrity. It is responsiveness to the moral costs of error; it is not fixed, static or unchangeable consistency. Integrity is not an abstract quality gifted to the great individual; it is culturally situated in social practices of responsibilities. To understand the influence of those on human transactions, practical and active reasoning is called for to perceive and reflect on these cultural practices. Ethical decisions do not just involve the person; they involve others, both in the present and in the future. Actions, and inaction, have consequences for us all. As 'ethical canary', the whistleblower signals this.

INTEGRITY AND THE CODES

In the professional and organizational life of health and social care, the concept of 'integrity' makes an appearance in the lexicon of professional codes of conduct. The word 'integrity', from the Latin *integritas*, means honesty, soundness and uprightness; it is 'wholeness' without any part removed or taken away. Thus defined, integrity coexists in these codes alongside standards that delineate, measure, quantify and evaluate chunks of health and soial care work. This is a curious recasting of a moral premiss into a prosaic parameter that can be safely measured and managed.

In her discussion of moral integrity in professional life, Banks (2010) set out three versions of what it is to act with moral integrity. First, she said integrity was the individual's conduct and compliance with their professional code of practice and rules of the profession; in other words, the actions of the professional. These professional codes set out rules of 'dos and don'ts', important insofar as they guide and give direction, but dangerous when those tasked with adhering to the rules become unthinking, and cease to question the impact of those rules on themselves or on people they are paid to care for, support or treat.

Second, Banks proposed that integrity could be understood as 'standing for something'; in other words, demonstrating commitment to particular principles and values in the social context within which the value of those commitments is referenced. The downside of this 'standing for something' is its individualization – that is, the individual is tasked with the commitment, but the situation and social context in which they are expected to deliver that commitment remain unexamined, thus rendering it unproblematic. The lone professional trying to work to deliver these principles and values may quickly burn out as they single-handedly address the superhuman task of attempting to resolve structural problems alone.

Third, Banks suggested that moral integrity was a capacity to reflect on and make sense of the dynamic nature of the world. This capacity is not the fixed structure of some 'good self', but it evolves and re-forms in light of experience. The context within which this capacity is exercised and made real itself requires critical examination.

For Banks, all three elements of integrity overlapped; they were not linear, sequential or either/or. This overlap is found in the social, political and professional cultures of health and social care. For the whistleblower, it is those cultures and its leaders, spared as they are from demands that they manifest, or are similarly infused with, 'integrity', which may pose the greatest threat to wrongs being righted.

As to what 'ethics' embraces, Banks (2014) suggested some or all of the following:

- conduct (what actions and behaviours are considered right or wrong)
- character (moral qualities viewed as good or bad)
- relationships (responsibilities attached to relationships between people, communities, with others)
- the 'good society' (where people are free and flourish harmoniously with other sentient beings in their shared natural environment).

In health and social care, burgeoning codes of conduct and statements of ethics typically narrow this list down, reductively, to conduct and the promotion of rights of people using these services (even though the resources necessary to realize those rights may be lacking), and people's exercise of choice (within limits). In doing this, these codes aim to prevent harm, rather than promote rights, care or goodness.

Codes of conduct and practice in health and social care do not set out features of any 'good society' or lay out any vision of how it might come to be. They seldom refer to the interpersonal, interactive nature of professional and social life. They mostly overlook power disparities and inequality, although international social work does stake out its professional terrain in human rights and social justice (IFSW 2014). In England and Wales, social care codes of conduct make statements about actions and behaviours (CCW 2015; HCPC 2016). These codes, insofar as they comprise ethical statements, are prescriptive. For example, the Code of Professional Practice for Social Care in Wales (CCW 2015, p.11) states 'you must act with integrity and uphold public trust and confidence in the social care profession'. This is followed by a series of prohibitions – what the worker must not do, rather than how they might act, including 'you must not abuse the trust of individuals…'; 'you must not directly or indirectly abuse, neglect or harm individuals, carers or colleagues…' The Code's requirements are thus framed in terms of individual actions and prohibitions. They decontextualize these from wider social relations, such as power and authority, inequality, social justice; as well as from organizational realities, such as resource availability and the calibre of the organization's leadership. The emphasis of this professional code of practice (and the codes of other health and care professions are similar) is on conformity to standards, and compliance with rules.

Meeting standards of practice is obviously necessary in health and social care, and it is not suggested that standards that are publicly and transparently agreed are anything other than a useful safeguard for citizens. But they are not the whole story, the *integritas* of practice. Those standards are found in their social and political surroundings; they are not absolutes, they evolve and change. Making a case for a situated ethics of social justice, Banks (2014) called for ethics to be positioned in the lives of people, in the realities and sensitivities of social situations and human relationships of which they are part. She located ethics in politicized social movements to promote social justice and human rights. Values embedded in this include moral courage, a 'quality or disposition to act in situations where such actions are difficult, uncomfortable or fear-inducing' (Banks 2014, p.20), or virtue, that speaks out against what is unjust, wrong or not right. This is whistleblowing by another name.

Seen this way, ethical practice is working with the contradictions and complexity of human life. It is a continual process of negotiating, appraising and weighing care, control, prevention, action, authoritative practice. Ethical practice is not just following rules; it is reflexively engaging with them to keep the point of the rules to the fore – the health, care and wellbeing of the other person. And ethical practice requires competence and courage, qualities often manifested by the whistleblower who speaks out about wrongdoing in health and social care. It is in this frame of reference that whistleblowing and raising concerns are situated.

WHISTLEBLOWING AS ETHICAL RIGHT ACTION

Many stories of whistleblowers – and there are increasing numbers of whistleblowers speaking out even as their careers are interred (Smith 2014) – illustrate recurrent themes. The familiar storyline here goes something like this: an employee noticed wrongdoing and tried to put it right. When this was unsuccessful, they raised their concerns with those who could do something to put them right. When this failed, and their concerns were ignored, the whistleblower tried again, and outside the immediate workplace situation. As their concerns continued to be ignored, the whistleblower found themselves scapegoated, bullied, threatened or victimized. Suffering professional and financial detriment, the whistleblower lost their job and, very likely, the possibility of working in their sector, workplace or profession, again.

The cases of two NHS doctors illustrate this, those of consultant doctors David Drew and Raj Mattu, as described in Chapter 5 (see page 98). David Drew, a consultant paediatrician in the English Midlands who raised concerns about a child safeguarding matter (the child died, aged 16 months) and about patient care – that is, the care and treatment of newborn babies and very sick children – was sacked.

In his book, Drew (2014) recounted how he raised safeguarding concerns about the child Kyle Keen, and about the very low air temperature in the ward for neonates and sick children. Drew's descriptions of babies wearing bonnets and wrapped in blankets supplied by their parents, themselves clothed in scarves, hats and outdoor clothes as they tried to keep their sick child warm around the clock in this hospital ward, located as it was in one of the richest countries in the world, were disquieting.

Before raising the concerns he did, Drew had to first of all *notice* what was going on. He had to *pay attention* to the sick and vulnerable children he was paid to look after. To care enough to treat those sick children (and to raise the concerns he did), Drew had to *respond* to the needs of those children. He had to display and act with *responsiveness* as the experienced clinician he was. And Drew had to be *competent* in his practice. He had to have the resolve, resilience and determination to keep on raising those concerns: to act, in other words, with *responsibility*.

Raj Mattu, a consultant cardiologist, again in the English Midlands but in a different locality, also raised concerns. He complained about the risk posed by overcrowding patient beds into spaces designed for four cardiology beds, not five as was the hospital's practice. Mattu was troubled that this overcrowding risked patient lives: safety was compromised if equipment, such as oxygen or mains electricity, could not reach that extra, fifth, bed.

In its 2001 review of this hospital, the CHI (Commission for Health Improvement, set up under the Health Act 1999 to review clinical governance in NHS bodies in England and Wales and carry out investigations of NHS health providers), had criticized 'the unacceptable risk to patients of putting five beds in bays designed for four'; and it reported that senior staff felt intimidated about reporting their concerns (CHI 2001, p.vi, p.vii). After the chief executive of the hospital's management body rejected the CHI findings, Dr Mattu made a protected disclosure under the UK whistleblowing law, PIDA. In the familiar pattern of these things, a counter-allegation of bullying was made against Mattu. He was suspended from his post. His employers re-engineered his public interest disclosures into employment matters, meaning they fell outside the protection afforded to whistleblowers by the Public Interest Disclosure Act, such as that is. Over 200 counter-allegations were made against Mattu, all of which, after eight years, were found to be false. Thirteen years after Mattu first raised his concerns, an employment tribunal (which itself had sat for six months) made Mattu an award for compensation (Campbell 2014).

AN ETHIC OF CARE

As with Drew, Mattu's responses to the situation he discovered involved his paying attention, or noticing; his caring enough to respect, respond and act; and his being competent to know what should or should not happen in those situations. Those features are ones which Fisher and Tronto (1990) located in their development of an ethic of care, where care was defined expansively as a 'species activity that includes everything that we do to maintain, continue and repair our "world" so we can live in it as well as possible, that includes our bodies, our selves and our environment, all of which we seek to interweave in a complex life-sustaining web' (Tronto 1993, p.103).

Fisher and Tronto put forward four elements in their ethic of care. Each can be identified in the cases of Drew and Mattu above, and of other whistleblowers across different sectors, not only health and social care.

1. The first element of an ethic of care that Fisher and Tronto set out was *attentiveness* – paying attention to what is happening, to the needs of the other, to the impacts of actions and inaction on another. In this moral framework, not attending, in these and other ways, is a moral failing.

2. The second element of an ethic of care is that of *responsibility*, that is, the ability to respond to the needs of others within the cultural norms and practices that pertain, rather than simply obeying rules, following orders, meeting procedural requirements.

3. The third element of an ethic of care, *competence*, is necessary to provide care and to take care of – incompetent care is a moral failing. Incompetent care is not care: it is incompetence.

4. The fourth moral element is *responsiveness*, of and between the caregiver and care-receiver. If we need care we are, at that moment, vulnerable. How our vulnerability is responded to is a moral matter, and with moral consequences.

Care, then, is action; it is relationship, and it is care with and for each other. 'Caring with' is not just the private, privatized caring for the self or immediate others. It means caring enough to stand up for others, to do so for the sake of justice and principle, whether or not one likes the other, agrees with them or will have any future connection with them. It is both personal and impersonal. Personal, because standing shoulder to shoulder with another is solidarity of meaning and recognition of shared humanity. Impersonal, because this requires our setting aside personal preferences, likes and dislikes, to ensure, safeguard and sustain the care and wellbeing of others, over time. It is not enough to say (in the oft-misrepresented words of the economist John Maynard Keynes) that 'in the long run we are all dead', as the actions and inactions of the present cast their shadow long into the future. Caring with and caring about means caring enough not to do more harm. It means caring for right action, caring enough to stop detriment to another (Tronto 1995). This is the action of a whistleblower.

Tronto (2010), then, regarded all forms of care, whether direct one-to-one care or the leadership and management of health or care institutions, as relational practices. As practices of relationship, they ask that we pay attention to their purpose and to the power relations within them. For Tronto, a caring institution is clear in its purposes, and in its articulation of a set of values that everyone understands and signs up to, both in what they do and how they do it (and not just what they say they do). A caring institution is pluralistic in response to human diversity; it is sensitive to difference between people, their needs and wishes.

Tronto (2010, p.163) identified a number of 'warning signs' that should alert us to poor functioning in health and care systems.

She was thinking about institutional care, but these warning signs throw light on organizational functioning and behaviour across wider health and care provision. Most readily recognized as places providing poor care are those infested by dehumanizing, callous and rigid practices. Not helping a hospitalized older person eat the meal placed just out of their reach; not ensuring that adequate hydration is provided for those who cannot drink without help; calling patients by their bed number or diagnosis or condition, and not by the their name, are but some of the casual denigrations that characterize an inversion of ethical care into 'un-care' and 'don't-care'.

Another warning sign for Tronto was the organization's approach to meeting health or care needs. When fixed, prescribed and given, rather than personal, negotiated, relational, changing and context-dependent, this red flag can quickly degenerate into a commodification of care. Commodified care is timed and standardized; it is not a process within any relationship of care. Once care is commodified, it creates scarcity, rationing and deficit-driven thinking. This too easily ends with the hideous pretence of 'care' that is the 15-minute slot, where a care worker on minimum wage is expected to prepare food, help an adult eat it, and then help them wash and dress (Leonard Cheshire Disability 2013). This degrades care to a basic subsistence level of existence. It boils care down to mere routines of activity, devoid of attentiveness, responsiveness, responsibility, and still less humanity.

Finally, it was a warning sign for Tronto when health or social care organizations, faced with a budget shortfall, *de facto* reduced care worker wages by cutting their working hours, or simply stopped paying them for travel time between one service user and the next (BBC 2015). We can safely assume that the care workers referred to in this BBC news report were not gifted with powers of time travel: they had to work, unpaid, in their own time to make up for intervals spent getting from one client to another. And it is a certain warning sign when the real reduction of care worker wages, by one means or another, takes place without any proportionate pay cut for those paid to lead or manage these services.

WHISTLEBLOWING AND THE EMPEROR'S CLOTHES

As Tronto (2010, p.165) observed 'When care givers find themselves saying that they care despite the pressures and requirements of the organization, the institution has a diminished capacity to provide good care.' Meaningless managerial mantras about 'doing more with less' expose the emperor's lack of clothes, for those who care to look. Without recognition of the reality of this for the cared-for as well as the caregiver, without the organizational and political space for deliberation and dispassionate scrutiny of the actual impacts – not the sanitized rhetoric of the unquestioned 'inevitability' of austerity and cash cutbacks, for example – then ethical care of the health and wellbeing of people and communities at a systemic, social and political level, is simply stargazing fantasy. And it is this that whistleblowers often speak to when they raise concerns.

Care-talk – and particularly ethic-of-care-talk – offers possibility of a paradigm shift in the territory occupied by the contractual obligations, standards, measurements and performance targets that riddle health and care service systems. Caring practice at the personal level, whether provided by people paid to care or by those providing it as an act of love, duty or assumed responsibility, is situated in organizational, cultural and social practices, rules, obligations. These are nested care arrangements: each layer or set of surroundings impacts on the other. Economically unequal and socially unjust societies have profoundly different impacts on the personal care relationship than those where care is shared, accepted as a personal and social obligation and freed from the tyranny of the market with its core assumptions of scarcity, whether of time, money or talent.

Responsibility is the second element of Tronto and Fisher's ethic of care. At a systemic or social level, its antonym, irresponsibility, is present in a political, wilful blindness to the impacts of social policy on particular sections of society. For example, in England and Wales cuts in housing benefit for claimants living in social housing deemed to have a spare bedroom – the so-called the 'bedroom tax'– has resulted in many tenants going without food and heating, selling belongings and falling into debt to make up the shortfall between the benefit they receive and the rent they pay (Power, Provan and Serle 2014). Irresponsibility is inevitable when complex lines of accountability and authority break up the *integritas* of health and social care service systems, as in privatized, marketized, fragmented health and care systems. What Tronto (2010) called privileged irresponsibility is the pretence that social results of manmade (*sic*) systems and structures, such as ageism, gender or race inequality, are 'natural'. When passively accepted like this, these structural social problems, far from demanding structural solutions, are simply air-brushed away. They become invisible. They are unconsidered, unquestioned; they are just the way of things. The whistleblower who says the emperor is without clothes, who draws attention to the outcomes of policies and practices that deliver harm, and sometimes death, to vulnerable people, as Drew and Mattu did, becomes the scapegoat, not the hero.

THE WHISTLEBLOWER AND AN ETHIC OF CARE

One objection to an ethic of care is its supposed weakness in providing a theoretical basis for moral reasoning and ethical decision making in health and social care, even though it serves well as a general objective or intention (Woods 2011). But an ethic of care offers rather more than that in the planning and delivery of health and care. The present author has used the four elements of Fisher and Tronto's ethic of care – attend/pay attention; respond; be competent, show responsiveness – in work with health and care staff and social workers, and with people who are using health and care services and with those who run them, and found these readily understood and recognized, as matters that matter. Rather than morality and ethics being perceived as rarefied abstractions, these elements make sense to people who are paid to provide health and care to others, and to those who have cared for, and been cared for by, others. *People get an ethic of care.* Tronto's ethic of care doesn't set ethics out there, but in *here*. It doesn't ostracize whistleblowers or those raising concerns as difficult, different or deranged, but as people who have noticed what others have also noticed without taking action, and in so doing have stepped outside peer or team norms, dared to be different, and marked out different territory. As we have seen, the costs on them of doing this can be life-changing, often for the worse.

EMBEDDING AN ETHIC OF CARE INTO HEALTH AND SOCIAL CARE PRACTICE AND SYSTEMS

Care, as ethical practice, takes into account relational dimensions of caring, not just the bald transaction between service and citizen that health and care may be reduced to. An ethic of care has utility and application across each domain of health and social policy, leadership and practice. It has been used conceptually to scrutinize the ethical credentials of social care policy (Sevenhuijsen and Švab 2004); to examine the changing nature of care responsibilities in and outside work (Williams 2001); and the meaning of care work to lay carers (Barnes 2006). Woods (2011) argued that there are few better examples of an ethic of care in practice than in nursing, where it guides the moral ideals and ethically-focused practice of competent and committed nurses, the interpersonal caring activities of nursing, and the ethical dimensions and underpinning of what is considered good nursing practice.

Woods (2011) illustrated how morally committed nurses demonstrated a distinct care ethic in their practice, not one that was a sterile, standard issue nursing code or medical and bioethical model. Woods found that attributes such as having appropriate nursing values and character, being personally involved, advocating for the other and delivering expert care, were closely connected to care-based ethics. Caring about someone involves an attitude, a feeling state of mind. For Woods, an ethic of care was found in situations defined, not in terms of rights and responsibilities, but in terms of relationships of care in a particular context. It is the humane – and human – counterbalance to dehumanized box-ticking that passes off as accountability, and to turning the blind eye on problematic practice, to make sure that target is hit, bulls-eye.

An ethic of care is not just for the health or social care practitioner who manifests care in spite of the care-less environment in which they may work. The strong justification for using an ethic of care throughout health and social care services and systems is that it provides a language and an architecture to talk about care and to speak out when harmful care is delivered (Barnes and Brannelly 2008). The four elements of an ethic of care – attentiveness, responsibility, competence and responsiveness – as well as trust, do not prescribe the procedures, standards, codes of guidelines. Rather, an ethic of care embraces fundamental human needs, in or outside health and social care services. These include the need to be listened to and understood; to have personal uniqueness understood and honoured; to have connection with others, not disconnection; and to be in relationship with people, not rules and standards (Barnes and Brannelly 2008).

ETHICS AND CARE THROUGHOUT HEALTH AND SOCIAL CARE SYSTEMS

To support health and care provision with an ethic of care, the organizational and wider policy and regulatory systems that surround it – the architecture – have to uphold its four elements of attentiveness, responsibility, competence and responsiveness. These provide the ethical bedrock for health and care delivery, and for the proper handling of concerns raised by a whistleblower. For it is in the breach – when a whistleblower raises concerns that don't look good for the organization – that we may see how ethical the credentials of health and social care systems really are.

To map out how an ethic of care might construct that architecture – the superstructure of health and social care systems – Table 7.1 sets out the four elements of an ethic of care, alongside three conceptual domains of health and social care systems. These conceptual levels are, first, the individual practitioner (for example doctor, nurse, social worker, social care worker) who delivers health and social care directly to the patient or user of the service. The second conceptual level is that of the organization that employs or contracts health or social care practitioners. Third is the wider political, regulatory and policy system within which health and social care organizations, and those they employ, function. These conceptual levels are not discrete or separate entities; each impacts on the other.

Table 7.1 Bedding elements of an ethic of care into health and social care

Level → Element of the care ethic ↓	Practitioner[1]	Organization[2]	System[3]
Attentiveness	Practitioner is alert to and attends to the needs of the person using health and social care services.	Organization pays attention to sustaining healthy organizational cultures that are intolerant of poor care, and of not speaking out.	Pays attention to the impact of sick and unhealthy organizational cultures on people who deliver, and who rely on, health and social care services.
Responsibility	Practitioner demonstrates an ability to respond to individual health or social care needs.	Organizational systems, structures and processes underscore rules as the means, not the end, of ensuring quality health and social care delivery.	Held to account for realistic resourcing of health and social care; for the dysfunctional impacts of targets and standards; and for effectiveness of whistleblowing statute and regulation.
Competence	Practitioner is skilled and demonstrably competent in their work, and emanates care in doing it.	Organizational leadership ensures that adequately resourced employees deliver competent health or social care.	Law, policy and regulation are fit for purpose, and resource first-class education and training of health and social care practitioners.
Responsiveness	Practitioner responds immediately to the person at risk of poor care. Practitioner routinely raises concerns and speaks out about poor care.	Organizational leadership responds in real time to problems of quality in health or social care delivery. Leaders model critical thinking: they expect reports of suboptimal practice; they are concerned if there are none.	Law, policy and regulation provides effective whistleblower protection, and sanctions or criminalizes retaliation against the whistleblower.

Developed from the original work of Fisher and Tronto (1990) and Tronto (1993), and adapted from the model presented initially by Ash (2015).

1 'Practitioners' are health and social care staff who deliver one-to-one health and social care; for example, doctors, nurses, social workers, social care workers.

2 'Organization' refers to the health or social care agency; for example, social services department, hospital, private regulated health and social care services.

3 'System' represents the overarching policy, regulatory and political context to health and social care delivery.

ATTENTIVENESS

Attentiveness is the first element of an ethic of care. At the direct, one-to-one health or caregiving level, the practitioner and professional acting with attentiveness would be alert to, and wholly focused upon, the needs of the person using their service. This is an obvious expectation of health and social care professionals and practitioners, and it is a registration requirement of professional codes of practice that regulate doctors, nurses, social workers and social care workers (CCW 2015; GMC 2014; NMC 2015).

Things aren't quite so straightforward at the organizational level. Manifesting organizational attentiveness to human need requires rather more than rules and procedures, necessary as they are. Organizations whose leadership walks the talk of 'paying attention' are ones that put the work into creating and sustaining healthy organizational cultures. These are cultures where people are expected to be attentive to the needs of the users of the service, and where, as a matter of course, employees raise concerns and are confident these will be attended to. These are organizations whose leaders pay attention to lesson-learning in real time, rather than months or years later after a public inquiry. They are attentive to how the needs of people using services they are paid to run are actually met. These are organizations that, authentically (and without the artifice of 'your opinion is important to us' when all other indicators clearly show it is not) pay close attention to what health and social care employees, patients and service users tell them about their services. These are organizations led by people who understand and expect employees to pay attention and raise concerns as necessary, because they know such concerns are often the early warning signs of potential system failure.

At the third, wider regulatory and political system level, paying attention to the quality of health and social care would embrace awareness and alertness to the negative, destructive impacts of defensive, rulebook-driven practice, and to the 'name, shame and blame' punishment regimes that riddle parts of the NHS and elsewhere. A policy and regulatory system working first and foremost from an ethic of care would pay close attention to why it was that one in five doctors subjected to fitness-to-practise investigations by the General Medical Council (the regulatory body for doctors licensed to practise in the UK) believed they were victimized after whistleblowing; to why 38 per cent of these felt they were bullied, and why over a quarter had over one month off work as a consequence (Bourne *et al.* 2015; Francis 2015). These are stark patterns calling for the *attention* of regulation and policy making, within an ethic of care, not ramping up the retribution regime that can be the fitness-to-practise investigations.

This wider system would pay very close attention and question why billions of pounds of public money might be spent clearing up messes created because the concerns of people working in health and care were not attended to earlier (Hammond and Bousfield 2011). Operating ethically, these would be regulators and policy makers who paid attention, and then acted to disincentivize health and social care organizations who use public money intended for patient care, to pay top-end legal fees to defend themselves against the whistleblower (Campbell 2014).

RESPONSIBILITY

The second element of the ethic of care is *responsibility*. Aside from ethical considerations, 'responsibility' is often used accusatorily, to apportion blame. Trying to pin blame on someone attempts to show the connection between *x* and *y* and, as a consequence, the harm suffered. Blame-finding (very different from NHS adverse incident reporting schemes) has little truck with understanding structural processes that constrain and influence people in complex webs of often unjust social structures. This blame-finding paradigm does not concern itself – it does not exhibit an ability to *respond* – when those with the greatest power get the greatest pay-off after things have gone wrong in a health or social care service.

Understood ethically, however, responsibility at the one-to-one level is better understood as an *ability*, a style or an approach of the health or care practitioner to *respond* to the needs of the patient or service users. At the organizational level, responsibility understood in this way would regard *rules as the means and not the end of good quality care.* These would be organizations whose leaders and cultures regarded a person raising concerns as acting with responsibility.

At the wider policy and regulatory system level, responsibility within an ethical frame would ensure realistic resourcing for health and social care organizations to discharge their responsibilities properly. This wider regulatory, policy or political system level would endorse organizations that encouraged shortcomings and 'near misses' in practice (Macrae 2014a), as these are organizations that take their ability to respond to failure very seriously, in real time and not just in the breach. This wider policy and regulatory systems would call to account health and social care organizations that throw money at silencing the whistleblower, by any legal means necessary, without checking if the unpleasant odour wasn't something deeply rotten in the state of the health or social care service.

COMPETENCE

Competence is the third element of an ethic of care. Like the other elements, this is obvious and easily understood at the individual level, the direct giving of health or social care. Competent staff are properly skilled to do the job, *and they demonstrate care when doing their work competently.*

At the organizational level, competence within this ethical frame includes leadership and management styles that are fit for purpose. These are organizational leaders and managers who are competent to comprehend that they are paid, first and foremost, to support high quality health and social care delivery. These are leaders who are acutely aware that a key feature of their job involves seeking out and listening carefully to what competent professionals tell them about standards of care. These are leaders who do not confuse their own, or the organization's competence, with the creation and servicing of complex, resource-devouring systems that collect masses of information but fail to interrogate it competently.

Competence, within an ethic of care and present at the wider policy and regulatory system level, would find regulators, politicians and policy makers reticent about over-claiming what regulation could achieve. Competent policy and regulation would be evidence-based, and take all steps to ensure that fit-for-purpose statute, regulation, education and training of health and social care staff and those paid to lead and manage health and care services were in place, and evolved as patient and citizen needs and expectations changed.

RESPONSIVENESS

Finally, the fourth element of an ethic of care is *responsiveness*. At the person-to-person level, the practitioner displaying responsiveness in this ethical frame is alert to the human dimensions of health and care, such as the need for connection, kindness, respect and compassion. Responsiveness at the organizational level will be apparent, for example, in organizations that live and breathe patient care, and who publicly and openly value staff and patients who draw attention to shortcomings in practice. These are organizations where managers and leaders get concerned when they *don't* hear concerns raised (within or without any procedures for reporting concerns), and are curious about why that is. They are sharp enough to know that no news is not always good news. They ask probing questions of the mass of data they collect, to find out about the present quality, standard and patient experience of the health and care they are paid to provide. They are organizations whose first reaction to a whistleblower is to listen intently, fact-find and assess; and not to pour public money into paying legal fees to quash the whistleblower, come what may.

A political, policy and regulatory level exhibiting responsiveness within this ethical frame would effectively demand that organizations listen to, support and act on the concerns of whistleblowers. This systemic level would place legislation on the statute book to criminalize those taking retaliatory action against whistleblowers, to mark out an ethical space where wilful blindness to wrongdoing, and organizational reprisal and revenge against those drawing attention to it, were put beyond the pale of right action in public life. Finally, and obviously, a wider health and social care system exhibiting an ethic of care would be led by people who, authentically, behaved in this way themselves. The following chapter considers what leadership (across all three domains of health and care systems discussed here) that is rooted in the four elements of an ethic of care might look like.

CHAPTER 8

ETHICAL LEADERSHIP AND WHISTLEBLOWING

If the four elements of an ethic of care – attentiveness, responsibility, competence and responsiveness – are to be designed into the wider political, policy and regulatory frameworks and the organizations that deliver health and social care, then ethical leadership is a fundamental feature of that design blueprint. How the whistleblower is responded to, what happens to them and the concerns they raise, casts a telling light on the ethical colours of the organization. If the whistleblower is speaking out against a backdrop of organizational silence, secrets and lies, then it is to the leadership of the organization, and those entities to whom chief executives of health and social care services report, that they speak. For these disclosures to be 'heard', authentically and ethically, requires attentiveness, an ability to respond and competence to deal ethically with the disclosures, and responsiveness to rectify the potential harm they signal, without doing more harm. This is a leadership that emanates from the four elements of an ethic of care.

This chapter discusses ethical elements of leadership in health and social care, in the organization and the wider policy-making and regulatory context. First, it considers the 'art' of leadership, and the dangers of 'romancing' the leader, that is, overlooking the influence followers and organizational culture have, reflexively, on leaders and styles of leadership. Second, dimensions and impacts of ethical leadership are discussed, and the influences of these on organizational cultures and the responses of those to the whistleblower. Third, the emotional intelligence of the ethical leader is considered. The chapter argues that awareness of self and others, and of the emotional climate in organizations (including their secrets, silence and lies) are hallmarks of an emotionally intelligent ethical leader, and one well positioned to deal, ethically, with disclosures a whistleblower makes.

THE ART OF LEADERSHIP

Hannah Arendt, political philosopher and rapporteur of the Nazi Albert Eichmann's trial in Jerusalem at the start of the 1960s, came to the view that our decisions about right or wrong depend on the company we keep (Arendt 2003). Our view of what is acceptable, unacceptable, of good and bad, are judgements made in a particular personal, social and historical space or context; social attitudes are shaped by social mores, and these change. Racist denigration of people of colour or people of difference was an unpleasant, yet tolerated, commonplace in 1950s Britain and US. Decades of struggle, speaking out and activism put some legal protection against victimization and harassment on grounds of race and ethnicity onto the statute book, and rendered most gross forms of abuse socially unacceptable and illegal. This change came about in large part because some people stood up and spoke out, again and again, and acted to challenge injustice and put pressure on public opinion and the political classes. Legislation outlawing the most egregious discrimination resulted.

This historic social and cultural change didn't directly emanate from a 'Leader', but it did need the leadership of many to speak out, keep on speaking out, and lead the change through action and example. The whistleblower can be the lone voice speaking out, acting alone, yet articulating concerns of others. The whistleblower speaks to the leadership of organizations in which they work and, when heard and when others support them, can catalyse action against wrongdoing. Such is the art of ethical leadership: paying attention, acting to respond, skilled and competent, and responsive to the need to do the right thing.

ROMANCING THE LEADER

It's a short call from saying leaders make a difference to the moral climate in an organization – for better or for worse – to their romanticization as saviours or messiahs. The 'romance of leadership' is shorthand to describe how leaders get headline billing in organization studies and leadership development programmes that single out leadership as the focal input to the functioning of groups and organizations (Meindl, Ehrlich and Dukerich 1985, p.330). If disaster occurs, great claims are made, and the search commences, for a transformational leader to put things right. A familiar political response to failing health and care organizations is to embark upon the search for the New Leader – the one who saves the service, transforms failure into achievement, all in the first year. This is a narrative of the heroic figure of myth or fairytale; the selfless slayer of dragons of corruption, poor practice and unethical endeavour.

These claims of the power of the Great Leader have a point, but miss a point. Leadership depends on followers, and the buy-in that employees make to the organizational purpose that the leader, and leadership team, articulate. Leaders influence the behaviour of others to achieve a purpose. The style, character and integrity of organizational leaders, whether in health and social care or anywhere else, impacts on how those organizations go about their business, and how the people employed in them experience their work. They particularly influence the response a whistleblower gets when they raise concerns.

Leaders front organizational culture, but they are not the organizational culture. Transforming an organizational culture into one that expects employees to speak out about poor practice, that takes these reports seriously, and which does not countenance retaliation, scapegoating or persecution of the whistleblower, is on the way to becoming an ethical entity.

Leaders are pivotal ethical influences, for better or for worse, on the organizational culture and people who work in it. They do this, knowingly or unknowingly (that is, with or without their own awareness), by modelling ethical right action, being observed, imitated or identified with, by others (Brown, Treviño and Harrison 2005). The behaviour of an employee's boss is amongst the strongest influences on their own ethical behaviour, to a greater extent than the employee's own moral frameworks, or the behaviour of their peers (Schminke *et al.* 2002). Leaders and their leadership teams determine the allocation of resources; they signal where organizational priorities and interests lie. What leaders give their attention to, what they commit resources to (in real time, real life, not lip-service, 140-character soundbites), is observed and understood by those around them. It shapes the climate and culture of the organization and how whistleblowers are responded to.

ETHICAL LEADERS

If leadership influences an organization's ethical climate, then ethical leadership is crucial in shaping organizations that act ethically, to do the right thing rather just than do things right. Ethical leadership has been defined by Brown, Treviño and Harrison (2005, p.120) as 'the demonstration of normatively appropriate conduct through personal actions and interpersonal relationships, and the promotion of such conduct to followers through two-way communication reinforcement, and decision making'. This definition doesn't necessarily add an ethical dimension to a standard definition of 'leadership'. The 'normatively appropriate conduct' referred to in this definition happens in a context: we can speculate that normatively appropriate conduct in global banking may be a different creature than that in health and social care, or so we might hope.

Various behaviours and attitudes characterize a 'moral person' and a 'moral leader' (the latter would struggle to exist without the former). Personal integrity, honesty, trustworthiness, care about people and the broader society, and someone who behaves ethically in and outside work feature on this checklist (Treviño, Brown and Hartman 2003; Treviño, Hartman and Brown 2000). These are leaders who are regarded by others as moral and ethical. In large entities like an NHS hospital or a local authority social services, most employees don't see or have much contact with leaders; the information, perceptions and reputations that filter down are mediated through many managerial layers and a lot of workplace stories of organizational life, whether fact or fantasy. Senior managers may regard themselves as good people, but shouldn't assume that others do.

Developing, supporting and sustaining ethical leadership isn't something that can be quickly rustled up in the management kitchen using this year's leadership cookbooks of clichés and motivational soundbites. Eisenbeiß and Giessner (2012) argued that there were three interacting influences on the development and maintenance of ethical leadership in organizations:

1. First were contextual characteristics – the big picture – such as a spirit of human rights in that society, and the wider cultural values of responsibility, justice and humanity.

2. Second were the characteristics of a particular professional sector or industry, such as its complexity, or its core purpose, be that money-making or health and caregiving to sick or vulnerable people.

3. Third were the internal characteristics of the organization, the working parts of the way the organization functions, such as its ethical infrastructure and the ethical behaviour of leadership and its peers.

In the first of these – wider social and cultural context – social learning theory suggests that ethical leadership will emerge and be more easily sustained in societies with a strong spirit of human rights. In such places people, including leaders and employees in organizations, are socially influenced to understand ethical right action as indispensable to leadership. The development and maintenance of ethical leadership stands on four meta values of trust: responsibility; justice; humanity; and transparency (Eisenbeiß and Giessner 2012). In the UK NHS, for example, the sector is complex and differentiated: the interests of pharmaceutical companies, political classes, patients, health campaigners, public health bodies, registered professionals and other staff, do not always align. According to Eisenbeiß and Giessner (2012), the more complex the organization, sector or entity, the more challenging it is to develop and sustain ethical leadership. That complexity includes the knowledge needed to understand the organizational environment, the degree of predictable change in it, and the availability of resources.

On these criteria, the UK NHS and social care operate in über-complicated environments. These highly complex surroundings face huge challenges from many quarters; leaders simply may not have the capacity to breathe ethical dimensions into every aspect of functioning. They don't have control over everything. The content of their ethical mandate, when set in opposition to the real world of pharmaceutical industry profit-making, a hostile political climate of privatization, 'doing more with less' and other mood-boards of public policy, set up a cognitive dissonance, or disconnect (Festinger 1962). Working for a public mandate of humanitarian endeavour in a context of inhumane or destructive behaviour results in stress, distress and failure. But if ethical leadership – and its *sine qua non*, a political and policy framework rooted in an ethic of care – authentically drive and support the humane goals of the organization, then such destructive behaviour can gain little traction in health and social care service systems working to manifest an ethic of care.

Leaders become attractive, credible and legitimate role models by engaging in behaviours that followers regarded as normatively appropriate and altruistic rather than selfish (Brown, Treviño and Harrison 2005). Direct communication between leaders and followers about ethical standards is a crucial dynamic in the social learning process: there is a lot of white noise in large organizations and ethics talk can struggle to be heard. For Brown *et al.* (2005), ethical leadership developed from a combination of integrity, high ethical standards, considerate and fair treatment of employees, and holding people accountable for their conduct. They found ethical leadership was positively related to considerate behaviour, fairness, honesty and trust in interactions between people across the organization. It was not associated with social desirability bias (trying to please others), cynicism, manufacturing perceptions of similarity (trying to be 'one of the boys/girls'), nor with punitive oversight or admonition by the leader. Ethical leaders, then, are those who walk the talk, practise what they preach, behave as ethical role models and use the rewards and sanctions at their disposal to achieve ethical purposes of work (Brown *et al.* 2005). They are fair, considerate and authentic.

Ethical role models are likely to be those an employee has worked with closely or had frequent contact with (Weaver, Treviño and Agle 2005). You can't follow an ethical role model if you only encounter them in the stylized theatre of set-piece meetings. In his account of his dismissal from Walsall Manor Hospital in England for raising concerns, consultant paediatrician David Drew (2014), recalled how few visits, expressions of interest or concern the managers who were to dismiss him made to the archaic facilities in which he and his team cared for newborn babies and sick young children. Managers, when detached from the realities of lives, health, care, sickness and death that are the core business of the NHS and social care services, are more likely to protect themselves from public scrutiny, political censure, naming and shaming. Smith (2015) observed that when that happens, the needs of staff and consumers become secondary because, intentionally or not, the management infrastructure runs the organization to protect itself from external criticism. These are not the actions of leadership that exhibits an ethic of care, nor one that is likely to welcome the whistleblower speaking out.

ETHICAL LEADERSHIP AND AN ETHICAL ORGANIZATIONAL CULTURE

What a leader pays attention to creates and reinforces organizational culture – more so than, say, the intermittent, short-lived intensity of regulatory inspections of health or social care (Dean 2014). How leaders react to critical incidents or crises sends a message to the workforce. The 'ethical climate' of everyday organizational life – the formal and informal behavioural control systems of leadership, the authority structures, reward systems, codes and policies, decision-making processes, ethical norms and peer behaviour that underpin activity in an organization – sets the tone for behaviours and actions expected. Leaders underestimate at their peril, the power of this ethical climate to influence employee behaviour. If employees perceive an organizational climate as benevolent, their commitment to it is greater (Cullen, Parboteeah and Victor 2003). Organizations with ethics codes that are lived and breathed, and which include leadership support and reward systems for ethical behaviour, have the largest deterrent to unethical conduct. A workplace climate focused wholly on self-interest is most strongly associated with unethical behaviour commitment (Treviño, Butterfield and Meabe 1998). In places without a strong ethical impulse, leaders of similar hue adapt to that milieu and those tacit expectations. Employees and leaders-in-the-making with a stronger ethical drive to they way they work, will leave. These are not positive conditions for expecting, still less encouraging, employees to speak out about poor care.

DESIGNING ETHICAL LEADERS

There is enough evidence to say ethical leadership is effective leadership. In places that are run on ethical principles, employees perform better, have more job satisfaction and are more willing to report problems (Brown *et al.* 2005), and to go the extra mile in their work (Toor and Ofori 2009). Ethical leadership inspires more effective teamwork and a more optimistic workforce (De Hoogh and Den Hartog 2008). Ethical leadership influences like behaviour throughout the layers of the organization (Mayer *et al.* 2009). This makes a difference, for the better, in health and social care. These are big deals.

Given the influence of the organizational culture on the behaviour of those who work in it, then making an ethical leader *in situ* rests on the putative leader and the culture of the organization they lead. Recruitment and selection methods using ethical case studies and discussions, as well as personality trait analysis, are business-as-usual ways to spot the ethical leader – but, as noted, character analysis is not a reliable indicator of how potential leaders will behave *in vivo* (any more than it is in identifying a potential whistleblower). Moral reasoning can be developed in leadership training programmes (Treviño 1992), but it needs practice, reinforcement and validation in an organizational culture that supports, not stifles, it. What happens in the workplace shapes the leader; the leader shapes the ethicality of that workplace. Having other ethical role models is a significant influence on leadership development. The internal infrastructure of policy, procedures, performance management, appraisal systems, on-the-spot direction and feedback, reward and promotion schemes, all tie into the culture that can create or destroy ethical leadership.

Unless these point in the same ethical direction, then the ethicality of leader and follower behaviour in the workplace is diminished.

EMOTIONAL INTELLIGENCE AND THE ETHICAL LEADER

Emotions can run high when a whistleblower raises concerns. Fear, denial, defensiveness, guilt, blame and anger are some of the powerful, primitive and destructive reactions unleashed. Unethical, punishing, blame-ridden organizational cultures grow, feed and thrive on secrets, silence, walking on by and passive compliance at any cost. The response of the organizational leadership to the whistleblower and to the whistleblowing disclosures sets the tone for the organizational fall-out that may follow. It is argued here that an ethical leadership style, drawing on the four elements of Tronto's ethic of care (attentiveness, responsibility, competence and responsiveness) is likely to respond to the disclosure, and to the whistleblower, in ways that are tuned into raw emotions unleashed, and to the need to take ethical right action in all the circumstances. This requires an emotional intelligence that can read the situation, understand its dynamics, and act morally to put things right, rather than react fearfully to quash the whistleblower by any means necessary.

'Emotional intelligence' (EI) was originally defined as 'the ability to monitor one's own and others' feelings, to discriminate among them, and to use this information to guide one's thinking and action' (Salovey and Mayer 1990, p.189). EI describes mental and affective processes involved in recognizing, using, understanding and managing one's own and others' emotional states to solve problems and manage behaviour. These are competencies, not personality traits. They are skills that cannot exist outside the social context in which they are played out (Salovey and Grewal 2005). EI is involved in the capacity to pick up emotions, assimilate emotion-related feelings, and to understand and manage the information those emotions contain or convey (Mayer, Caruso and Salovey 1999).

For ethical leaders striving to manifest an ethic of care, and to bed a care ethic into the organization, EI would seem to be a prerequisite. EI does not elevate agreeableness – fitting in, conforming, keeping quiet about problems – over anything else (Mayer 2004). EI isn't a slew of happy-clappy motivational checklists or management mantras. EI is not emotional incontinence, overwrought emoting or emotivism. EI brings emotions (always present, mostly unattended to) and intelligence together. EI is a means whereby ethical right action, including speaking out about wrongdoing, occurs as a routine feature of organizational life. Leadership capacity and the ability to perceive and manage the emotional states of self and others, to understand the signs and signals extant in the organizational climate, are competencies that support the growth of an ethic of care in the organization. Genuine EI – that is, decoupled from personal aggrandisement, and wholly committed to ethical behaviour – combines being a moral manager, leader or employee, with being a moral person (Treviño *et al.* 2000). Behaving ethically requires a leader to ask routinely of themselves and others: would this action be seen as trustworthy by a reasonable observer? By a hostile media?

EI is cultivated with, and in relationship to, others. EI is relational; its development, practice and strengthening come about in interaction with others. Objectifying, action planning and running courses on EI that take the person out of the workplace merely reify and falsify the trait. EI cannot exist in a vacuum, it is situational. EI cannot be dislocated from the environment in which it exists. Stripping the person from the scenes of their life to train EI into them on a short course, risks losing the potential for moral depth. A calculating character, intent on 'using' EI for personal advancement or to boost their own bottom line, can quickly contrive the superficial trappings of EI in the training room (Culham and Bai 2011). What matters in the organization striving towards EI and an ethic of care is what happens in it day-in, day-out in the work people do to deliver health and social care.

EMOTIONAL INTELLIGENCE IN THE WORKPLACE

Increasing EI capacity may well rest on the cultivation and practice of compassion, courage, honesty and wisdom, traditionally regarded as virtue ethics. People who are in relationships that are not informed by morality may treat the other instrumentally – as a way of getting to where they want to be, by any means necessary (MacIntyre 2007). These are not behaviours that safeguard health and care services from wrongdoing, and still less challenge it when it occurs. Instead, imprinting ethical dimensions into work makes it more possible to realize an organizational culture that is emotionally intelligent, which is not consumed by, nor habituated to, base emotions of fear, anger, blame, denial and grief: those subjective, primitive emotions that are contagious, infectious and occasionally deadly in their impact on organizational health. People with high EI are more adept at reasoning through the emotional backcloth and precursors of their own behaviour and that of others. They have the capacity to use this constructively to guide their own and thinking and action. Organizational leaders with high EI appear more able to figure out – to read – the ethical or unethical behaviour of others. Overall, EI is predictive of individual ethicality and that of others. Employees with high EI have been found to be less likely than their low EI counterparts to interpret unethical behaviour of others as an excuse for their own. They don't follow the crowd, or take the line of least resistance. They appear also to have a stronger sense of integrity (Mesmer-Magnus *et al.* 2008). These are qualities to be nurtured and validated in organizations providing health and social care. They are often the qualities the whistleblower demonstrates.

EI has the potential to be a moral practice, and to sustain organizations embracing the four elements of an ethic of care, from top to bottom. Following Culham and Bai (2011), there are a number of ways EI, and the four elements of an ethic of care, might be hard-wired into the what and the how of the organization's work. These include:

1. defining the organization's purpose in terms of the four elements of an ethic of care, and working to realize each of these at each and every level of organizational hierarchy

2. growing leaders who, authentically, walk, live, breathe an ethic of care, and do so with emotional intelligence

3. providing *in vivo* support and development for EI, for contemplative practice on the four elements of an ethic of care,

for working with and through difficulties, and for speaking out about wrongdoing.

These are achievable goals when an organization commits to thinking about and understanding what an ethic of care means for their work. They are realizable when the leadership and the culture of the organization (which evolves reflexively) support and sustain these practices. But they are not achievable in organizations that regard morality and ethical endeavour as an instrumental other, to be bought in, measured, assessed, performance-managed, or used to demand 'doing more with less'. That is business as usual repackaged and tied up with a pretty, but wholly fake, moral bow.

CHAPTER 9

THE ETHICAL POINT OF WHISTLEBLOWING

Why have whistleblowers Julian Assange, Edward Snowden, Hervé Falciani of the HSBC bank and myriad others before them, had to leave their job and country? Why have NHS whistleblowers described in this book, and elsewhere (for example, Hammond and Bousfield 2011), been put through the purgatory that followed their speaking out about harm? This book set out to dig deeper into the dynamics of the phenomenon that is whistleblowing in health and social care. Its core premiss has been this: unless and until we understand and are prepared to face some uncomfortable truths about how we – collectively – tacitly condone this way of reacting to dissent and disclosure by staying silent, then whistleblowers, whether in the NHS, social care or any other sector, will go on facing the same stitch-ups when they raise their head above the parapet. As Smith (2015) commented, '…the NHS is not the problem, it is merely one symptom of a much broader pestilence'.

The book has argued that such 'pestilence' is rooted in the political, regulatory and organizational context of health and social care. The organizational dynamics of group and peer pressures to fit in and not be thought of as a troublemaker; public policy exigencies that routinize, standardize and measure what can be counted, rather than what counts for the person using those services, profoundly influence the creation of the organizational cultures and climates that are so often implicated, and sometimes complicit, in the wrongdoing that whistleblowers speak out about. If the whistleblower is the ethical canary in the organizational coalmine, then, for sure, the safety of the pit needs considerably more care and attention.

Hence the call here for an ethic of care to be embedded in the policy, regulation, leadership and delivery of health and social care. An ethic of care requires – throughout that system – *attentiveness* to human need; *responsibility* for right action, not only rules; the *competence* to provide the best health and care possible within an ethic of care; and *responsiveness* to the needs of the person requiring health or social care.

Organizational cultures uphold the ethical infrastructure of health or social care provision, for better or for worse. They do this within the policy and regulatory framework (and this includes resourcing) that pertains at the time. To attempt to frontload an ethic of care onto the organization, the profession or the service, without any attention to the intended and unintended impacts of these policy and regulatory frameworks on ethical practice, is futile. Simplistically superimposing, for example, an ethical code of practice onto the health and social care organization (inevitably setting up another compliance hoop for the employee to jump through), on top of supra-organizational practices, and policy and regulatory demands that are themselves devoid of any ethicality, merely overfeeds organizational cultures already bloated with cynical, robotic box-ticking. There has to be another way.

LEADERSHIP, ANTI-BATHSHEBA STYLE

Developing an ethical culture ingrained with an ethic of care throughout the health and social care system calls – at its simplest and at its most challenging – for a change of emphasis from the leader as the 'Great Person', to a leader as reflective human being. If leadership is (at least in part) modelling, then qualities of reflection, the capacity to pay attention to and think about ethical health and caregiving, to take responsibility and not to buck-pass, blame or cover up, to ensure health and social care organizations and their policy and regulatory framework are competent, fit for purpose and responsive to the needs of people who depend on them, are core competencies of a new type of emotionally intelligent leadership that may spring from an ethic of care. This is a new, ethical leadership for the *integritas* of the health and social care system: policy, regulation and delivery.

Leaders of the 'Great Person' command-and-control school of leadership, who are paid wildly more than most people they employ, who are shielded from the everyday working life of the people they lead, who will likely never experience the needs of the people who use the service, easily fall prey to the 'Bathsheba Syndrome' (Ludwig and Longenecker 1993) – they simply will not get it: the trappings, perks and privileges they enjoy as leaders (whether as politicians, permanent secretaries, chief executives, directors or other elevated positions within the system that is health and social care), where their phone calls are returned, their emails answered and firewalled, where they have use of resources and enjoy benefits denied others, and where they hold the (false) belief that they can control events or circumstances, insulate them from the exigencies, trade-offs and compromises that others routinely find themselves making to deliver the service the Bathsheba Syndrome leader leads, and about which the whistleblower raises concerns.

Health and social care systems urgently need to weed out – nip in the bud – the creation of any more leaders of the Bathsheba Syndrome tendency. Instead, the imperative is to cultivate what we might call 'Anti-Bathsheba' leadership, the leader who works with, in and from an ethic of care. Anti-Bathsheba leaders, whether they occupy the political, policy-making, regulatory or organizational wings of health and social care systems, would be those who make sure they are surrounded by critical friends in their leadership team, people who are curious and who question, who add reason and reasoning, who can ask hard questions of hard data, and do so from outside the comfort of conventional wisdom and the herd mentality. Anti-Bathsheba would be the leader who regards saying 'I don't know' as a mark of integrity, not ineptitude. Anti-Bathsheba would ask, and pay close attention to, what employees say about the organization, and they would not shoot, or arrange for others to shoot, the messenger when they are told. They are the antithesis of the 'Great Person' school of leadership and its autocratic, organizational cultures that regard criticism as disloyalty, and which traduce the one speaking out as the troubling and troubled 'not a team player'. In social work, for example, Anti-Bathsheba would be concerned that UK social work professionals are, by and large, *uncritical*, that is, unquestioning, of the organizational cultures and structures in which they practise (Preston-Shoot 2010). Anti-Bathsheba would understand how such passive, docile behaviour impacts, and not healthily, on the value of a critical, questioning social work practice. And Anti-Bathsheba is conscious of the power they hold to value and validate those who question, challenge and think.

Anti-Bathsheba would resist stress and pressure themselves, and avoid subjecting others to it for prolonged periods. They know stress disinhibits: when people are tired, exhausted or hungry, right action and right decision making are jeopardized. Long working hours deplete ego and cognitive controls on behaviour; that moral muscle loses its strength (Brown and Mitchell 2010). People become too exhausted to speak out about anything. Anti-Bathsheba is not afraid to call to account those whose ethical behaviour falls short, and expects others to call them out if they act outside an ethic of care. They lead organizations where people (inside or outside it) have confidence that unethical behaviour will come to light, and be penalized when it does.

Anti-Bathsheba would recognize, as research has consistently done, that whistleblowers are not mentally ill, disgruntled or deranged troublemakers; but instead would understand whistleblowing as a prosocial, positive act of significant potential benefit to the organization. Far from adding to '21 ways to skin a whistleblower' (Bousfield 2011), Anti-Bathsheba would lead from the front to stop reprisals, threats or vexatious complaints to a regulator about the whistleblower (just three of those 21 ways), and instead would regard whistleblowing as providing a constructive internal warning light. These are leaders who recognize that while smiling, compliant yes-men and yes-women seem easier to manage (they always go along with the mainstream), it's the extroverts with low agreeableness, the non-drones, those whose first priority is to the profession and people it serves, rather than to the bureaucracy that surrounds (or stifles) it, who are the ones to cultivate in any leadership team and workforce. Anti-Bathsheba knows that it is fear of retaliation, and of the consequences of being seen to grass up colleagues, that keeps people quiet. Anti-Bathsheba recognizes that their emotionally intelligent leadership of open organizational cultures, where doubts are expressed and listened to, can antidote this (de Graaf 2010).

ANTI-BATHSHEBA AND LEARNING THOSE LESSONS

'Learning lessons' has featured several times in this book. There is a lot of happy talk about organizations learning lessons after disasters in health and social care, rather in the mould of the penitent who periodically seeks absolution, only to fall immediately back into the same unthinking behaviour. To learn from failure is a process. It is a practice that needs practice. It is the corrective to an escalation of commitment to harmful action, where the intensity of doing the same wrong things over and over again increases after each failure (Sleesman *et al.* 2012). Failure can be big or small: an organization's ability to learn from failure is best measured in how it deals with a range of large and small outcomes that deviate from what's expected or desired, rather than focusing only on how it handles major disasters (Cannon and Edmondson 2005). The Anti-Bathsheba leader knows that learning isn't a trade-marked technique to be trotted out when the chips are down. Anti-Bathsheba pays attention to small deviations from what is expected, whether to the good or the bad, and shapes an organizational culture where people develop the skill, and get the practice, of *learning*.

Barriers to learning are bedded into, sometimes buried in, the way the organization goes about its work. There is a strong personal and social reaction against being seen to fail, or acknowledging failure. Again, it is the whistleblower who may be that voice off that says things are not as they appear. Being seen as successful has huge social *cachet* for leaders of the old style Bathsheba Syndrome persuasion. Managers have an incentive to distance themselves from failure. Organizational procedures and policies, and senior management, can discourage people from trying things out and failing, especially when those organizations work in highly politicized environments of health and social care that are under perpetual public gaze. Shared learning is a risky business; hot emotions emerge and many old school Bathsheba Syndrome leaders aren't able to handle these. Social and cognitive systems tend to shut down analysis of failure. People feel negative emotions when exposing their own failures, and may lack the competencies to do so, which are detachment, dispassionate interest, and separation of the self from the failure. Carrying out any effective examination of failure requires patience, and tolerance of mess, uncertainty and not knowing. This doesn't fit, at all, with political demands for action yesterday, blame, for yes/no, did he/didn't he (*sic*) answers, all with the accompanying familiars ('lessons have been learned') of action plans and checklists. The comfort of self-confirming beliefs is a much more alluring place to stay (Cannon and Edmondson 2005).

If the futile drive is for learning only from 'success', then failure will follow (Baumard and Starbuck 2005). Anti-Bathsheba would reframe failure as 'learning' or 'practice', and regard it as an inevitable, everyday, to-be-expected part of complex, skilled and demanding human services work. Trite presentational tat like 'zero tolerance' can be ditched when health and social care systems start to learn. Accountability for critical thinking, for thinking through what is done and why, for asking good questions, for probing, interrogating and constantly seeking to understand and improve, can replace risk-averse, defensive, box-ticking compliance.

Anti-Bathsheba leaders are inquisitive. They value the critical thinker and the whistleblower. Anti-Bathsheba leaders recognize that danger lurks when only like-minded people talk to each other, remembering that groups of similars tend to end up in a more extreme position after discussion than where they were before it (Sunstein 2014). Anti-Bathsheba leads by not countenancing the closing-off and convenient collapse into consensus, without deep penetration of the matter in hand, and from within an ethic of care. Anti-Bathsheba wants, expects and, when they step forward with concerns, listens very carefully to whistleblowers.

THE VIRTUE OF WHISTLEBLOWING

Egan (1994), when talking about the shadow side of organizations, said it took competence and guts to deal with the undiscussables of organizational life. The whistleblower names these undiscussables when they speak out. In doing this, they counteract powerful, covert pressures of silence and denial at work which ensure the undiscussable stays exactly that. They bring wrongdoing to light. Virtue that may be, but unrewarded it mostly remains.

Health and social care systems built on and operating with an ethic of care front, centre and throughout their work, need the whistleblower. More wrongdoing is uncovered by whistleblowers, across all sectors, than by any of the apparatus that is audit, the media, regulators, management and cyber-paper chase accoutrements of organizational life (Evans 2008). Whistleblowing may bring to light illegal or unethical activity (Vadera, Aguilera and Caza 2009; Warren 2003). When the whistleblower raises concerns, the organization has the chance to self-correct a problem, outside of the public and political gaze. It has the opportunity to deliver on its paper policies and handle the disclosures decently and ethically. In acting this way, the organization sets up a virtuous circle. It signals its intolerance of wrongdoing, its valuing of the whistleblower, and its right action to put wrong right.

Working within and from an ethic of care, health and social care organizations and their policy makers and regulators should not fear whistleblowers. They should encourage and welcome them. Cultivating and nurturing organizational cultures where people speak out about poor practice before it gets normalized, is the counterbalance to harm and the slippery slope that leads to disasters. This is the culture of Anti-Bathsheba leadership in health and social care, where whistleblowing is recognized not as a threat, but as means of ensuring that the best possible health and social care is available to people who need it.

POSTSCRIPT FOR THE WHISTLEBLOWER

This book did not set out to provide a 'how to' manual for the whistleblower, nor for the employer they disclose to. Its purpose has been to wake up the worlds of health and social care, from politicians, policy makers and regulators, to care workers and ward orderlies, to powerful dynamics of organizational life that are mostly covert, hidden or ignored, until the whistleblower turns the light on wrongdoing. If it achieves that, then the book's work is done.

But in a spirit of mitigating any disappointment a whistleblower-in-the-making may be feeling that they've been short-changed, here are some suggestions and some advice. It is not legal advice, just the learning of one who has walked this path, and more than once. Others may give you different counsel. Listen to it.

1. First, having read this book you must disabuse yourself of any false belief that you will be hailed as the hero for doing your job when you speak out to disclose a public interest concern. If this happens, your story needs to be told, and the culture and ethicality of your employer publicized, widely, for others to see. Health and social care need more employers like this.

   Instead, expect, and plan for, the strong possibility that you will come under the organization's investigatory spotlight. Is your family prepared for this? Do your loved ones understand what you're speaking out about and why? Do they care enough to care for you while you go through this? Are you prepared for the very real possibility that long-term friends and colleagues will evaporate when you call on them for support? Read up on others' experiences of whistleblowing before you disclose. Whistleblower Wendy Addison's experiences and blog at www.speakout-speakup.org are worth looking at. There are some very useful practical handbooks for the whistleblower, such as Australian Brian Martin's *Whistleblowing: A Practical Guide* (2013; free to download), and Tom Devine and Tarek Maassarani's (2011) *The Corporate Whistleblower's Survival Guide*, which has a US focus. There are NGOs working with whistleblowers internationally, the Whistleblowing International Network (a global coalition of organizations with experience advising whistleblowers: www.whistleblowingnetwork.org) and Transparency International, working to give voice to the victims and witnesses of corruption (www.transparency.org).

2. Before you make any decision about disclosing, get your facts, dates, times, observations about your concern written down. Detail, detail, detail. Be aware that writing this down at work carries its own risks, so think carefully about the best place to do this. Anything you write or send from work to your home, or elsewhere, is traceable. Be aware that if you have employer documents at home or elsewhere, you may be accused of theft down the line. If you can, wait until you've had professional, preferably legal, advice (see 4 below) before accumulating corroborative material off-site, and be very careful if you do.

3. Check out your concerns with others at work. Have you got this right? Is there another, benign and plausible, explanation? If not, will others stand up to speak out with you? If so, they are your allies. However, having read this book, you will not be surprised if support ebbs away when you try to call it up.

4. Get professional, preferably legal, advice. Consult your country's whistleblowing NGO if you have one. In the UK, the charity PCaW will advise potential whistleblowers raising public interest concerns. Make sure you understand what protection you have in law, and what your employer's whistleblowing procedures demand of you. Find out what corroborative information you need, and how you can protect

yourself against any future accusations of theft of material or maleficence, for example. Understand, before you make your disclosure, how you can protect yourself from counter-allegations and accusations that may be thrown at you. What's the worst thing the employer can say about you? Think worst-case scenarios and get prepared. None of us is perfect, so get your reasoning clear, and your ducks in a row. Be proactive. Think ahead.

5. Understand that your trade union may or may not be your friend, if and when you seek its advice about making a public interest disclosure. Some trade unions and professional bodies lie very close to the employer. This may not be to your benefit. If it is, then that will be valuable support.

6. Make sure your lawyer or trade union representative earns your trust. Don't just give it. Satisfy yourself that your lawyer or trade union rep is skilled, competent and experienced in supporting whistleblowers, understands the law, and is on your side, not the employer's. Ask them how many whistleblowing cases they have dealt with, with what outcome. Ask them what you can expect from them. Over and above that, your lawyer or representative needs to *earn* your trust. Don't trust others to support you unless and until they demonstrate to you that they are worthy of that trust, and that they are competent and committed to look after you, the whistleblower.

REFERENCES

Adams, G.B. and Balfour, D.L. (1998) *Unmasking Administrative Evil*. Thousand Oaks, CA: Sage Publications.

Aitkenhead, D. (2013) 'NHS chief, David Nicholson: 'I've never been ashamed of anything I've done'.' *The Guardian*, 19 July.

Aldrich, H.E. and Ruef, M. (2006) *Organizations Evolving*. (Second edition). Thousand Oaks, CA: Sage Publications.

Alford, C.F. (2001) *Whistleblowers. Broken Lives and Organisational Power*. Ithaca, NY: Cornell University Press.

Anand, V., Ashforth, B.E. and Joshi, M. (2004) 'Business as usual: The acceptance and perpetuation of corruption in organizations.' *Academy of Management Executive 18*, 2, 39–53, doi:10.5465/ame.2004.13837437

Arendt, H. (1963) *Eichmann in Jerusalem. The Banality of Evil*. New York: Viking.

Arendt, H. (2003) *Responsibility and Judgement*. New York: Schocken Books.

Argyris, C. (1980) 'Making the undiscussable and its undiscussability discussable.' *Public Administration Review 40*, 3, 205–213.

Argyris, C. (1986) 'Skilled incompetence.' *Harvard Business Review 64*, 5, 74–79.

Argyris, C. (1990) *Overcoming Organizational Defenses: Facilitating Organizational Learning*. Boston, MA: Allyn and Bacon.

Armenakis, A. (2004) 'Making a difference by speaking out: Jeff Wigand says exactly what's on his mind.' *Journal of Management Inquiry 13*, 4, 355–362.

Ash, A. (2010) 'Ethics and the street level bureaucrat: Implementing policy to protect elders from abuse.' *Ethics and Social Welfare 4*, 2, 201–209.

Ash, A. (2011) 'A culture of complicity.' *Community Care*, 31 March.

Ash, A. (2013) 'A cognitive mask? Camouflaging dilemmas in street level policy implementation to safeguard older people from abuse.' *British Journal of Social Work 43*, 1, 99–115.

Ash, A. (2014a) *Safeguarding Older People from Abuse. Critical Contexts to Policy and Practice*. Bristol: The Policy Press.

Ash, A. (2014b) 'Safeguarding Older People from Mistreatment. Social Work's Ethical Dilemmas and an Ethic of Care.' In S. Hessle (ed.) *Human Rights and Social Equality: Challenges for Social Work*, Vol.1. Farnham: Ashgate.

Ash, A. (2015) 'Whistleblow or Walk on By? Ethics and Cultures of Collusion in Health and Social Care.' In D. Lewis and W. Vandekeckhove (eds) *Developments in Whistleblowing Research 2015*. London: International Whistleblowing Research Network.

Ashforth, B.E. and Anand, V. (2003) 'The normalization of corruption in organizations.' *Research in Organizational Behavior 25*, 1–52.

Attree, M. (2007) 'Factors influencing nurses' decisions to raise concerns about care quality.' *Journal of Nursing Management 15*, 392–402.

Bandura, A. (1999) 'Moral disengagement in the perpetuation of humanities.' *Personality and Social Psychology Review 3*, 3, 193–209.

Bandura, A. (2008) 'Reconstrual of "Free Will": From the Agentic Perspective of Social Cognitive Theory.' In J. Baer, J.C. Kaufman and R.F. Baumeister (eds) *Are We Free? Psychology and Free Will.* Oxford: Oxford University Press.

Banks, S. (2010) 'Integrity in professional life: Issues of conduct, commitment and capacity.' *British Journal of Social Work 40*, 7, 2168–2184.

Banks, S. (2014) 'Ethics.' In I. Ferguson and M. Lavalette (eds) *Critical and Radical Debates in Social Work.* Bristol: Policy Press.

Barnes, M. (2006) *Care and Social Justice.* Basingstoke: Palgrave Macmillan.

Barnes, M. and Brannelly, T. (2008) 'Achieving care and social justice for people with dementia.' *Nursing Ethics 15*, 3, 384–395.

Bauman, Z. (1989) *Modernity and the Holocaust.* Ithaca, NY: Cornell University Press.

Bauman, Z. (1993) *Postmodern Ethics.* Oxford: Blackwell.

Bauman, Z. (2000) 'Am I my brother's keeper?' *European Journal of Social Work 3*, 1, 5–11.

Baumard, P. and Starbuck, W.H. (2005) 'Learning from failures: Why it may not happen.' *Long Range Planning 38*, 3, 281–298.

Baumeister, R.F. and Leary, M.R. (1995) 'The need to belong: Desire for interpersonal attachments as a fundamental human motivation.' *Psychological Bulletin 117*, 3, 497–529, doi:10.1037/0033-2909.117.3.497

Bazerman, M.H. and Banaji, M.R. (2004) 'The social psychology of ordinary ethical failures.' *Social Justice Research 17*, 2, 111–115.

Bazerman, M.H. and Tenbrunsel, A.E. (2012) *Blind Spots: Why We Fail to Do What's Right and What to Do about It.* Princeton, NJ: Princeton University Press.

BBC (2011) 'Undercover reporter "haunted" by abuse of patients.' *Panorama* programme broadcast on 31 May. Accessed on 19 August 2015 from www.bbc.co.uk/panorama/hi/front_page/newsid_9501000/9501531.stm.

BBC (2015) 'Care workers "not given enough travel time" between jobs.' BBC News. Available at www.bbc.co.uk/news/uk-wales-south-west-wales-32031538, accessed on 7 April 2016.

Bocchiaro, P., Zimbardo, P.G. and Van Lange, P.A.M. (2012) 'To defy or not to defy: An experimental study of the dynamics of disobedience and whistle-blowing.' *Social Influence 7*, 1, 35–50.

Bourne, T., Wynants, L., Peters, M., Van Audenhove, C., Timmerman, D., Van Calster, B. *et al.* (2015) 'The impact of complaints procedures on the welfare, health and clinical practice of 7926 doctors in the UK: A cross-sectional survey.' *BMJ Open 5*, doi: 10.1136/bmjopen-2014-006687

Bousfield, A. (2011) '21 ways to skin an NHS whistleblower.' Accessed on 20 March 2015 from http://medicalharm.org/uncategorized/the-full-21-ways-to-skin-a-whistleblower.

Bouville, M. (2008) 'Whistle-blowing and morality.' *Journal of Business Ethics 81*, 3, 579–585.

Bowen, F. and Blackmon, K. (2003) 'Spirals of silence: The dynamic effects of diversity on organizational voice.' *Journal of Management Studies 40*, 6, 1393–1417.

Brown, A.J. (2008) *Whistleblowing in the Australian Public Sector: Enhancing the Theory and Practice of Internal Witness Management in Public Sector Organisations.* Canberra: Australian National University Press.

Brown, M.E. and Mitchell, M.S. (2010) 'Ethical and Unethical Leadership.' *Business Ethics Quarterly 20*, 4, 583–616.

Brown, M.E., Treviño, L.K. and Harrison, D.A. (2005) 'Ethical leadership: A social learning perspective for construct development and testing.' *Organizational Behavior and Human Decision Processes 97*, 2, 117–134.

Burger, J.M. (2009) 'Replicating Milgram: Would people still obey today?' *American Psychologist 64*, 1, 1–11.

Campbell, D. (2014) 'Whistleblowing heart doctor who aired hospital safety fears wins tribunal case.' *The Guardian*, 17 April. Accessed on 17 October 2015 from www.theguardian.com/society.

Cannon, M.D. and Edmondson, A.C. (2005) 'Failing to learn and learning to fail (intelligently): How great organizations put failure to work to innovate and improve.' *Long Range Planning 38*, 3, 299–319.

Carroll, E. (2015) 'Working as a mental health nurse in today's NHS drained me of compassion.' *The Guardian*, 17 August. Accessed on 17 August 2015 from www.theguardian.com.

Casey Report (2015) *Report of Inspection of Rotherham Metropolitan Borough Council.* London: Department for Communities and Local Government. HC1050.

CCW (Care Council for Wales) (2015) *Code of Professional Practice for Social Care.* Cardiff: Care Council for Wales.

Cesarani, D. (2005) *Eichmann: His Life and Crimes.* London: Vintage.

CHI (Commission for Health Improvement) (2001) *Clinical Governance Review. University Hospitals Coventry and Warwickshire NHS Trust.* London: The Stationery Office.

Chugh, D., Bazerman, M.H. and Banaji, M.R. (2005) *Bounded Ethicality as a Psychological Barrier to Recognizing Conflicts of Interest.* Cambridge: Cambridge Books Online.

Cohen, S. (2001) *States of Denial. Knowing about Atrocities and Suffering.* Cambridge: Polity Press.

Culham, T. and Bai, H. (2011) 'Emotional intelligence meets virtue ethics: Implications for educators.' *Journal of Thought*, Fall/Winter, 25–43.

Cullen, J.B., Parboteeah, K.P. and Victor, B. (2003) 'The effects of ethical climates on organizational commitment: A two-study analysis.' *Journal of Business Ethics 46*, 2, 127–141.

Darley, J.M. and Latané, B. (1968) 'Bystander intervention in emergencies: Diffusion of responsibility.' *Journal of Personality and Social Psychology 8*, 4, Part1, 377–383.

Davies, N. (2014) *Hack Attack. How the Truth Caught Up with Rupert Murdoch.* London: Chatto and Windus.

Davis, K. and Frederick, W.C. (1984) *Business and Society: Management, Public Policy, Ethics.* New York, NY: McGraw Hill.

de Graaf, G. (2010) 'A report on reporting: Why peers report integrity and law violations in public organizations.' *Public Administration Review*, September/October, 767–779.

De Hoogh, A.H.B. and Den Hartog, D.N. (2008) 'Ethical and despotic leadership, relationships with leader's social responsibility, top management effectiveness and subordinates' optimism: A multi-method study.' *The Leadership Quarterly 19*, 297–311.

De Maria, W. (2006) 'Common law – common mistakes? Protecting whistleblowers in Australia, New Zealand, South Africa and the United Kingdom.' *International Journal of Public Sector Management 19*, 7, 643–658.

Dean, A. (2014) 'How to survive a CQC inspection.' *Guardian Professional*, 4 August. Accessed on 4 August 2014 from www.theguardian.com.

Devine, S. and Devine, T. (2010) *Whistleblower Witch Hunts: The Smokescreen Syndrome.* Washington DC: Government Accountability Project.

Devine, T. and Maassarani, T.F. (2011) *The Corporate Whistleblower's Survival Guide. A Handbook for Committing the Truth.* San Francisco: Berrett-Koehler Publishers.

Dozier, J.B. and Miceli, M.P. (1985) 'Potential predictors of whistle-blowing: A prosocial behavior perspective.' *The Academy of Management Review 10*, 4, 823–836.

Drew, D. (2014) *Little Stories of Life and Death @NHSwhistleblowr.* Leicester: Matador.

Egan, G. (1994) *Working the Shadow Side: A Guide to Positive Behind-the-Scenes Management.* San Francisco: Jossey-Bass.

Ehrlinger, J., Gilovich, T. and Ross, L. (2005) 'Peering into the bias blind spot: People's assessments of bias in themselves and others.' *Personality and Social Psychology Bulletin 31*, 5, 680–692.

Eisenbeiß, S.A. and Giessner, S.R. (2012) 'The emergence and maintenance of ethical leadership in organizations.' *Journal of Personnel Psychology 11*, 1, 7–19.

Evans, A.J. (2008) 'Dealing with dissent: Whistleblowing, egalitarianism, and the republic of the firm.' *Innovation. The European Journal of Social Sciences 21*, 3, 267–279.

Festinger, L. (1962) 'Cognitive dissonance.' *Scientific American, 207*, 4, 93–107.

Fisher, B. and Tronto, J.C. (1990) 'Toward a Feminist Theory of Caring.' In B. Fisher (ed.) *Circles of Care: Work and Identity in Women's Lives.* Albany, NY: SUNY Press. Cited in J.C Tronto 'Creating caring institutions.' *Ethics and Social Welfare 4*, 2, 158–171.

Fotaki, M. (2014) 'Can consumer choice replace trust in the National Health Service in England? Towards developing an affective psychosocial conception of trust in health care.' *Sociology of Health And Illness 36*, 8, 1276–1294.

Fotaki, M. and Hyde, P. (2015) 'Organizational blind spots: Splitting, blame and idealization in the National Health Service.' *Human Relations 68*, 3, 441–462.

Francis, R. (2013a) *Report of the Mid Staffordshire NHS Foundation Trust Public Inquiry.* Volumes 1–3. London: The Stationery Office. HC 898-I. 6 February.

Francis, R. (2013b) *Report of the Mid Staffordshire NHS Foundation Trust Public Inquiry. Executive Summary.* London: The Stationery Office. HC 947. 6 February.

Francis, R. (2013c) *Chairman's Press Statement. Mid Staffordshire NHS Foundation Trust Inquiry.* www.midstaffspublicinquiry.com. 6 February.

Francis, R. (2015) *Freedom to Speak Up. An Independent Review into Creating an Open and Honest Reporting Culture in the NHS.* www.gov.uk/government/publications/sir-robert-francis-freedom-to-speak-up-review. Report published 11 February 2015.

Gere, J. and MacDonald, G. (2010) 'An update of the empirical case for the need to belong.' *Journal of Individual Psychology 66*, 1, 93–115.

Glazer, M.P. and Glazer, P.M. (1989) *The Whistleblowers. Exposing Corruption in Government and Industry.* New York, NY: Basic Books Inc.

Giddens, A. (1990) *The Consequences of Modernity.* Cambridge: Polity Press.

Gino, F. and Bazerman, M.H. (2009) 'When misconduct goes unnoticed: The acceptability of gradual erosion in others' unethical behaviour.' *Journal of Experimental Social Psychology 45*, 708–719.

GMC (General Medical Council) (2014) *National Training Survey 2014. Bullying and Undermining.* Accessed on 10 May 2015 from www.gmc-uk.org/NTS_bullying_and_undermining_report_2014_FINAL.pdf_58648010.pdf.

Goffman, E. (1974) *Frame Analysis. An Essay on the Organization of Experience.* Cambridge, MA: Northeastern University Press.

Goldie, J., Schwartz, L., McConnachie, A. and Morrison, J. (2003) 'Students' attitudes and potential behaviour with regard to whistle blowing as they pass through a modern medical curriculum.' *Medical Education 37*, 268–375.

Grant. C. (2002) 'Whistle Blowers: Saints of Secular Culture.' *Journal of Business Ethics 39*, 391–399.

Grover, S.L. and Hui, C. (2005) 'How job pressures and extrinsic rewards affect lying behaviour.' *International Journal of Conflict Management 16*, 3, 287–300.

Greenberger, D.B., Miceli, M.P. and Cohen, D.J. (1987) 'Oppositionists and group norms: The reciprocal influence of whistle-blowers and co-workers.' *Journal of Business Ethics 6*, 7, 527–542.

Hammond, P. (2015) *Staying Alive: How to Get the Best from the NHS*. London: Quercus.

Hammond, P. and Bousfield, A. (2011) 'Shoot the messenger. How NHS whistleblowers are silenced and sacked.' *Private Eye*, Issue 1292, 8–22 July.

Harrison, S. and Smith, C. (2004) 'Trust and moral motivation: Redundant resources in health and social care.' *Policy and Politics 32*, 3, 371–386.

HCPC (Health & Care Professions Council) (2016) *Standards of Conduct, Performance and Ethics*. London: HCPC.

Hedin, U. and Månsson, S. (2012) 'Whistleblowing processes in Swedish public organisations – Complaints and consequences.' *European Journal of Social Work 15*, 2, 151–167.

Heffernan, M. (2011) *Wilful Blindness*. London: Simon and Schuster.

HOC (House of Commons) Committee of Public Accounts (2014) *Whistleblowing*. Ninth Report of Session 2014–15. HC593. London: Stationery Office.

HOC (House of Commons) Health Committee (2015) *Complaints and Raising Concerns*. HC 350. London: The Stationery Office, 21 January.

Holt-Lunstad, J., Smith, T.B., Baker, M., Harris, T. and Stephenson, D. (2015) 'Loneliness and social isolation as risk factors for mortality: A meta-analytic review.' *Perspectives on Psychological Science 10*, 2, 227–237.

Hughes, D. (2013) 'NHS hospitals spend £2m on gagging orders preventing staff speaking out.' *The Independent*, 12 June.

Humphrey, C. (2015) 'Face-to-face: Social work and evil.' *Ethics and Social Welfare 9*, 1, 35–50.

Hunton, J.E. and Rose, J.M. (2011) 'Effects of anonymous whistle-blowing and perceived reputation threats on investigations of whistle-blowing allegations by audit committee members.' *Journal of Management Studies 48*, 1, 75–98.

IFSW (International Federation of Social Workers) (2014) *Global Definition of Social Work*. Approved by the IFSW General Meeting and the IASSW General Assembly, July. Available at http://ifsw.org/get-involved/global-definition-of-social-work/, accessed on 21 March 2016.

Ingersoll, V.H. and Adams, G.B. (1992) *The Tacit Organization*. Greenwich, CT: JAI Press.

Jackson, D., Peters, K., Hutchinson, M., Edenborough, M., Luck, L. and Wilkes, L. (2011) 'Exploring confidentiality in the context of nurse whistleblowing: Issues for nurse managers.' *Journal of Nursing Management 19*, 655–663.

Jay Report (2014) *Independent Inquiry into Child Sexual Exploitation in Rotherham 1997–2013*. Accessed on 2 September 2014 from www.rotherham.gov.uk/inquiry.

Jones, A. and Kelly, D. (2014) 'Whistle-blowing and workplace culture in older peoples' care: Qualitative insights from the healthcare and social care workforce.' *Sociology of Health and Illness 36*, 7, 986–1002.

Jos, P.H., Tompkins, M.E. and Hays, S.W. (1989) 'In praise of difficult people: A portrait of the committed whistleblower.' *Public Administration Review 49*, 6, 552–561.

Jubb, P.B. (1999) 'Whistleblowing: A restrictive definition and interpretation.' *Journal of Business Ethics 21*, 1, 77–94.

Kaptein, M. (2008) 'Developing and testing a measure for the ethical culture of organizations: The corporate ethical virtues model.' *Journal of Organizational Behavior 29*, 7, 923–947.

Keenan, J.P. (1990) 'Upper-Level Managers and Whistleblowing: Determinants of Perceptions of Company Encouragement and Information About Where to Blow the Whistle.' *Journal of Business and Psychology 5*, 2, 223–235.

Kennedy, I. (2001) *The Report of the Public Inquiry into Children's Heart Surgery at the Bristol Royal Infirmary 1984–1995: Learning from Bristol.* (Cm 5207) London: The Stationery Office. 18 July.

Kiesler, C.A. and Kiesler, S.B. (1969) 'Group Pressure and Conformity.' In J. Mills (ed.) *Experimental Social Psychology.* New York, NY: Macmillan.

King's Fund (2014) *Culture and Leadership in the NHS. The King's Fund 2014 Survey.* London: The King's Fund.

Lacayo, R. and Ripley, A. (2002) 'Persons of the Year. The whistleblowers.' *Time Magazine,* 30 December.

Latané, B. and Darley, J.M. (1968) 'Group inhibition of bystander intervention in emergencies.' *Journal of Personality and Social Psychology 10*, 3, 215–221.

Leonard Cheshire Disability (2013) 'Ending 15-minute care.' www.leonardcheshire.org.

Lewis, D. (2008) 'Ten years of public interest disclosure legislation in the UK: Are whistleblowers adequately protected?' *Journal of Business Ethics 82*, 497–507.

Lewis, D. (2010) 'Introduction.' In D.B. Lewis (ed.) *A Global Approach to Public Interest Disclosure. What Can we Learn from Existing Whistleblowing Legislation and Research?* Cheltenham: Edward Elgar Publishing.

Lewis, D. (2011) 'Whistleblowing in a changing legal climate: Is it time to revisit our approach to trust and loyalty at the workplace?' *Business Ethics: A European Review 20*, 1, 71–87.

Lewis, D., Brown, A.J. and Moberly, R. (2014) 'Whistleblowing: Its Importance and the State of the Research.' In A.J. Brown, D. Lewis, R.E. Moberly and W. Vandekerckhove (eds) *International Handbook on Whistleblowing Research.* Cheltenham: Edward Elgar Publishing.

Lewis, D., D'Angelo, A. and Clarke, L. (2015) *The Independent Review into Creating an Open and Honest Reporting Culture in The NHS. Quantitative Research Report. Surveys of NHS Staff, Trusts and Stakeholders.* London: Middlesex University.

Lifton, R.J. (1986) *The Nazi Doctors: Medical Killing and the Psychology of Genocide.* New York: Basic Books.

Lucy, D., Poorkavoos, M. and Wellbelove, J. (2014) *The Management Agenda 2014.* Horsham: Roffey Park Institute.

Ludwig, D.C. and Longenecker, C.O. (1993) 'The Bathsheba Syndrome: The ethical failure of successful leaders.' *Journal of Business Ethics 12*, 265–273.

MacIntyre A. (2007) *After Virtue. A Study in Moral Theory.* (Third edition). Notre Dame, IN: University of Notre Dame Press.

Macrae, C. (2014a) 'Early warnings, weak signals and learning from healthcare disasters.' *BMJ Quality and Safety Online First, 23*, 440–445.

Macrae, C. (2014b) *Close Calls.* Basingstoke: Palgrave Macmillan.

Mansbach, A. (2011) 'Whistleblowing as Fearless Speech: The Radical Democratic Effects of Late Modern Parrhesia.' In D. Lewis and W. Vandekeckhove (eds) *Whistleblowing and Democratic Values.* London: International Whistleblowing Network.

Marshak, R.J. (2006) *Covert Processes at Work: Managing the Five Hidden Dimensions of Organisational Change.* San Francisco: Berrett-Koehler Publishers.

Martin, B. (2013) *Whistleblowing: A Practical Guide.* Sparsnäs, Sweden: Irene Publishing.

Mayer, J. (2004) 'Be Realistic.' *Harvard Business Review 82*, 28.

Mayer, J.D., Caruso, D. and Salovey, P. (1999) 'Emotional intelligence meets traditional standards for an intelligence.' *Intelligence 27*, 267–298.

Mayer, D.M., Kuenzi, M., Greenbaum, R., Bardes, M. and Salvador, R. (2009) 'How low does ethical leadership flow? Test of a trickle-down model.' *Organizational Behavior and Human Decision Processes 108*, 1, 1–13.

Mead, N.L., Baumeister, R.F., Gino, F., Schweitzer, M.E. and Ariely, D. (2009) 'Too tired to tell the truth: Self-control resource depletion and dishonesty.' *Journal of Experimental Social Psychology, 45*, 3, 594–597.

Meindl, J.R., Ehrlich, S.B. and Dukerich, J.M. (1985) 'The romance of leadership.' *Administrative Science Quarterly 30*, 1, 78–102.

Mesmer-Magnus, J., Viswesvaran, C., Joseph, J. and Deshpande, S.P. (2008) 'The role of emotional intelligence in integrity and ethics perceptions.' *Research on Emotion in Organizations, 4*, 225–239.

Miceli, M.P. (2004) 'Whistle-blowing research and the insider: Lessons learned and yet to be learned.' *Journal of Management Inquiry 13*, 4, 364–366.

Miceli, M.P. and Near, J.P. (1985) 'Characteristics of organizational climate and perceived wrongdoing associated with whistle-blowing decisions.' *Personnel Psychology 38*, 525–544.

Miceli, M.P. and Near, J.P. (1992) *Blowing the Whistle: The Organizational and Legal Implications for Companies and Employees.* New York, NY: Lexington Books.

Miceli, M.P. and Near, J.P. (2005) 'Standing up or standing by: What predicts blowing the whistle on organizational wrongdoing?' *Research in Personnel and Human Resources Management 24*, 95–136.

Miceli, M.P., Near, J.P. and Dworkin, T.M. (2008) *Whistle-Blowing in Organizations.* New York: Routledge.

Miceli, M.P., Near, J.P. and Dworkin, T.M. (2009) 'A word to the wise: How managers and policy-makers can encourage employees to report wrongdoing.' *Journal of Business Ethics 86*, 379–396.

Miceli, M.P., Near, J.P., Rehg, M.T. and Van Scotter, J.R. (2012) 'Predicting employee reactions to perceived organizational wrongdoing: Demoralization, justice, proactive personality, and whistle-blowing.' *Human Relations 65*, 8, 923–954.

Mid Staffordshire NHS Foundation Trust Inquiry (2010) Independent Inquiry into Care Provided by Mid Staffordshire NHS Foundation Trust. January 2005–March 2009 (Vol.1). London: The Stationery Office. HC375-I Session 2009/10.

Milgram, S. (1974) *Obedience to Authority. An Experimental View.* New York: Harper and Row.

Milliken, F.J. and Morrison, E.W. (2003) 'Shades of silence: Emerging themes and future directions for research on silence in organizations.' *Journal of Management Studies 40*, 6, 1563–1568.

Moore, D.A. and Loewenstein, G. (2004) 'Self-interest, automaticity, and the psychology of conflict of interest.' *Social Justice Research 17*, 2, 189–202.

Morrison, E.W. and Milliken, F.J. (2000) 'Organizational silence: A barrier to change and development in a pluralistic world.' *Academy of Management Review 25*, 4, 706–725.

Moscovici, S. (1976) *Social influence and social change.* London: Academic Press.

Moscovici, S. (1980) 'Toward a Theory of Conversion Behavior.' In L. Berkowitz (ed.) *Advances in Experimental Social Psychology* (Vol. 13, pp.209–239). New York, NY: Academic Press.

Moscovici, S., Lage, E. and Naffrechoux, M. (1969) 'Influence of a Consistent Minority on the Responses of a Majority in a Color Perception Task.' *Sociometry 32*, 4, 365–380.

Moscovici, S. and Zavalloni, M. (1969) 'The group as a polarizer of attitudes.' *Journal of Personality and Social Psychology 12*, 2, 125–135, doi:10.1037/h0027568

Muehlheusser, G. and Roider, A. (2008) 'Black sheep and walls of silence.' *Journal of Economic Behaviour and Organization 65*, 387–408.

Near, J.P. and Miceli, M.P. (1985) 'Organizational dissidence: The case of whistleblowing.' *Journal of Business Ethics*, 4, 1–16.

Near, J.P. and Miceli, M.P. (1995) 'Effective whistle-blowing.' *Academy of Management Review* 20, 3, 679–708.

Near, J.P. and Miceli, M.P. (1996) 'Whistle-blowing: Myth and reality.' *Journal of Management* 22, 3, 507–526.

Near, J.P. and Miceli, M.P. (2011) 'Integrating Models of Whistle-Blowing and Wrongdoing: A Proposal for a New Research Agenda.' In J. Jetten and M. Hornsey (eds) *Rebels in Groups: Dissent, Deviance, Difference and Defiance.* Oxford: Blackwell-Wiley.

Near, J.P., Rehg, M.T., Van Scotter, J.R. and Miceli, M.P. (2004) 'Does type of wrongdoing affect the whistle-blowing process?' *Business Ethics Quarterly 14*, 2, 219–242.

NMC (Nursing and Midwifery Council) (2015) *The Code. Professional Standards of Practice and Behaviour for Nurses and Midwives.* London: Nursing and Midwifery Council.

Noelle-Neumann, E. (1974) 'The spiral of silence. A theory of public opinion.' *Journal of Communication 24*, 2, 43–51.

Noonan, W.R. (2007) *Discussing the Undiscussable: A Guide to Overcoming Defensive Routines in the Workplace.* San Francisco, CA: Jossey-Bass.

OPCW (Older People's Commissioner for Wales) (2012) *Raising Concerns in the Workplace.* Cardiff: OPCW.

PAC (Public Accounts Committee) (2014) *Oral Evidence: Whistleblowing. Ninth Report of Session 2014–15.* HC 1117: www.publications.parliament.uk/pa/cm201415/cmselect/cmpubacc/593/593.pdf. 24 March. Available to view at www.parliamentlive.tv/Event/Index/7d285e74-9371-4441-8411-9bca742fbed7.

Pattenden R. (2003) *The Law of Professional–Client Confidentiality. Regulating the Disclosure of Confidential Personal Information.* Oxford: Oxford University Press.

Perry, N. (1998) 'Indecent exposures: Theorizing whistleblowing.' *Organization Studies 19*, 2, 235–257.

PCaW (Public Concern at Work) (2013) *The Whistleblowing Commission. Report on the Effectiveness of Existing Arrangements for Workplace Whistleblowing in the UK.* London: PCaW, November.

Peirce, E., Smolinski, C.A. and Rosen, B. (1998) 'Why sexual harassment complaints fall on deaf ears.' *Academy of Management Executive 12*, 3, 41–54.

Pemberton, S., Tombs, S., Chan, M.M.J. and Seal, L. (2012) 'Whistleblowing, organisational harm and the self-regulating organisation.' *Policy and Politics 40*, 2, 263–279.

Pinder, C.C. and Harlos, K.P. (2001) 'Employee silence: Quiescence and acquiescence as responses to perceived injustice.' *Research in Personnel and Human Resources Management 20*, 331–369.

Power, A., Provan , B. and Serle, N. (2014) *The Impact of Welfare Reform on Social Landlords and Tenants.* York: Joseph Rowntree.

Preston-Shoot, M. (2010) 'On the evidence for viruses in social work systems: Law, ethics and practice.' *European Journal of Social Work 13*, 4, 465–482.

Ramesh, R. (2013) 'NHS chief denies cover-up over £2m gagging orders.' *The Guardian*, 2 June.

Rehg, M.T., Miceli, M.P., Near, J.P. and Van Scotter, J.R. (2008) 'Antecedents and outcomes of retaliation against whistleblowers: Gender differences and power relations.' *Organization Science, 19*, 221–240.

Rest, J.R. (1986) *Moral Development: Advances in Research and Theory.* New York: Praeger.

Rothschild, J. and Miethe, T. (1999) 'Whistle-blower disclosures and management retaliation.' *Work and Occupations 26*, 1, 107–128.

Salovey, P. and Grewal, D. (2005) 'The science of emotional intelligence.' *Current Directions in Psychological Science 14*, 6, 281–285.

Salovey, P. and Mayer, J.D. (1990) 'Emotional intelligence.' *Imagination, Cognition, and Personality 9*, 185–211.

Schein, E.H. (2010) *Organizational Culture and Leadership* (Fourth edition). San Francisco, CA: John Wiley & Sons.

Schminke, M., Wells, D., Peyrefitte, J. and Sebora, T.C. (2002) 'Leadership and ethics in work groups: A longitudinal assessment.' *Group and Organization Management 27*, 2, 272–293.

Schneider, B. and Barbera, K.M. (2014) 'Introduction.' In B. Schneider and K.M. Barbera (eds) *The Oxford Handbook of Organizational Climate and Culture*. Oxford: Oxford University Press.

Sevenhuijsen, S. and Švab, A. (2004) *The Heart of the Matter*. Ljubljana: Peace Institute, Institute for Contemporary Social and Political Studies.

SGASB (South Gloucestershire Safeguarding Adults Board) (2012) *Winterbourne View Hospital. A Serious Case Review*. Accessed on 3 March 2013 from www.southglos.gov.uk/wv/report.pdf. http://sites.southglos.gov.uk/safeguarding/adults/i-am-a-carerrelative/winterbourne-view.

Sims, R.L. and Keenan, J.P. (1998) 'Predictors of external whistleblowing: Organizational and intrapersonal variables.' *Journal of Business Ethics 17*, 411–421.

Skivenes, M., and Trygstad, S.C. (2010) 'When whistle-blowing works: The Norwegian case'. *Human Relations 63*, 7, 1071–1097.

Sleesman, D.J., Conlon, D.E., McNamara, G. and Miles, J.E. (2012) 'Cleaning up the big muddy: A meta-analytic review of the determinants of escalation of commitment.' *Academy of Management Journal 55*, 3, 541–562.

Smith, A. (2014) "There were hundreds of us crying out for help': The afterlife of the whistleblower.' *The Guardian*, 22 November. Accessed on 10 December 2015 at www.theguardian.com/society/2014/nov/22/there-were-hundreds-of-us-crying-out-for-help-afterlife-of-whistleblower.

Smith, A. (2015) 'We need to protect whistleblowers outside the NHS too.' *The Guardian*, 12 February. Accessed on 12 February 2015 at www.theguardian.com/commentisfree/2015/feb/2012/protect-whistleblowers-outside-nhs-too-francis-review.

Smith, M. (2011) 'Reading Bauman for social work.' *Ethics and Social Welfare 5*, 1, 2–17.

Stansbury, J.M. and Victor, B. (2009) 'Whistle-blowing among young employees: A life-course perspective.' *Journal of Business Ethics 85*, 281–299.

Staub, E. (1989) *The Roots of Evil. The Origins of Genocide*. Cambridge: Cambridge University Press.

Staub, E. (1999) 'The roots of evil: Social conditions, culture, personality, and basic human needs.' *Personality and Social Psychology 3*, 3, 179.

Sunstein, C.R. (2014) *Conspiracy Theories and Other Dangerous Ideas*. New York, NY: Simon & Schuster.

Sunstein, C.R. and Hastie, R. (2015) *Wiser: Getting Beyond Groupthink to Make Groups Smarter*. Boston, MA: Harvard Business Review Press.

Tajfel, H., Billig, M.G., Bundy, R.P. and Flament, C. (1971) 'Social categorization and intergroup behaviour.' *European Journal of Social Psychology 1*, 2, 149–178.

Tenbrunsel, A.E. and Messick, D.M. (1999) 'Sanctioning systems, decision frames, and cooperation.' *Administrative Science Quarterly 44*, 4, 684–707.

Tenbrunsel, A.E. and Messick, D.M. (2004) 'Ethical fading: The role of self-deception in unethical behavior.' *Social Justice Research 17*, 2, 223–236.

Tenbrunsel, A.E., Diekmann, K.A., Wade-Benzoni, K.A. and Bazerman, M.H. (2010) 'The ethical mirage: A temporal explanation as to why we are not as ethical as we think we are.' *Research in Organizational Behavior 30*, 0, 153–173.

Tenbrunsel, A.E., Smith-Crowe, K. and Umphress, E.E. (2003) 'Building houses on rocks: The role of the ethical infrastructure in organizations.' *Social Justice Research 16*, 3, 285–307.

The Guardian (2014) 'Rebekah Brooks email on Tony Blair advice.' *The Guardian*, 19 February 2014. Accessed on 16 September 2014 from www.theguardian.com/uk-news/interactive/2014/feb/19/rebekah-brooks-email-tony-blair-advice-pdf.

The Guardian (2015) 'Lack of support for whistleblowers is a disgrace.' *The Guardian*, 15 February 2015. Accessed on 15 February 2015 from www.theguardian.com/society/2015/feb/15/whistleblowers-should-law-punish-hospital-bosses.

Toor, S. and Ofori, G. (2009) 'Ethical leadership: Examining the relationships with the Full Range Leadership Model, employee outcomes, and organizational culture.' *Journal of Business Ethics Quarterly 90*, 533–547.

Toynbee, P. (2015) 'Who dares confront Jeremy Hunt, NHS bully-in-chief?' *The Guardian*, 17 February.

Treviño, L.K. (1992) 'The social effects of punishment in organizations: A justice perspective.' *Academy of Management Review 17*, 647–676.

Treviño, L.K. and Youngblood, S.A. (1990) 'Bad apples in bad barrels: A causal analysis of ethical decision-making behaviour.' *Journal of Applied Psychology 75*, 4, 378–385.

Treviño, L.K., Brown, M. and Hartman, L.P. (2003) 'A qualitative investigation of perceived executive ethical leadership: Perceptions from inside and outside the executive suite.' *Human Relations 55*, 5–37.

Treviño, L.K., Butterfield, K.D. and Meabe, D.M. (1998) 'The ethical context in organizations: Influences on employee attitudes and behaviors.' *Business Ethics Quarterly 8*, 447–476.

Treviño, L.K., Hartman, L.P. and Brown, M. (2000) 'Moral Person and Moral Manager: How Executives Develop a Reputation for Ethical Leadership.' *California Management Review 42*, 4, 128–142.

Treviño, L.K., Weaver, G.R. and Brown H. (2008) 'It's lovely at the top: Hierarchical levels, identities, and perceptions of organizational ethics.' *Business Ethics Quarterly 18*, 2, 233–252.

Treviño, L.K., Weaver, G.R. and Reynolds, S.J. (2006) 'Behavioral ethics in organizations: A review.' *Journal of Management 32*, 6, 951–990.

Tronto, J.C. (1993) *Moral Boundaries: A Political Argument for an Ethic of Care.* New York: Routledge.

Tronto, J.C. (1995) 'Care as a basis for radical political judgments.' *Hypatia 10*, 2, 141.

Tronto, J.C. (2010) 'Creating caring institutions: Politics, plurality and purpose.' *Ethics and Social Welfare 4*, 2, 158–171.

Tronto, J.C. (2013) *Caring Democracy. Markets, Equality, and Justice.* New York: New York University Press.

Tsahuridu, E.E. (2011) 'Whistleblowing Management is Risk Management.' In D. Lewis and W. Vandekerckhove (eds) *Whistleblowing and Democratic Values.* London: International Whistleblowing Research Network.

Tsahuridu, E.E. and Vandekerckhove, W. (2008) 'Organisational whistleblowing policies: Making employees responsible or liable?' *Journal of Business Ethics 82*, 1, 107–118.

Vadera, A.K., Aguilera, R.V. and Caza, B.B. (2009) 'Making sense of whistle-blowing's antecedents: Learning from research on identity and ethics programs.' *Business Ethics Quarterly 19*, 4, 553–586.

Vandekerckhove, W. (2011) 'Five Paradoxes in Managing Whistle-blowing.' Paper given at *Speak-Up Procedures* conference. University of Greenwich, London, 4 October.

Vandekerckhove, W. (2012) *Public Support for Whistleblowers.* London: University of Greenwich Business School. Accessed on 11 May 2015 from http://ssrn.com/abstract=2176193.

Vandekerckhove, W. (2014) 'Virtue ethics and management.' Accessed on 3 May 2015 from www.academia.edu/6225582/Virtue_ethics_and_management.

Vandekerckhove, W. and Rumyantseva N. (2014) *Freedom to Speak Up – Qualitative Research.* London: University of Greenwich, 19 November.

Walker, G. (2015) *Letter to Rt Hon Jeremy Hunt MP.* 6 March. Accessed on 12 November 2015 at www.garywalker.org.uk.

Walker, M.U. (2007) *Moral Understandings.* (Second edition). New York: Oxford University Press.

Warren, D.E. (2003) 'Constructive and destructive deviance in organizations.' *Academy of Management Review 28,* 4, 622–632.

Weaver, G.R., Treviño, L.K. and Agle, B. (2005) 'Somebody I look up to: Ethical role models in organizations.' *Organizational Dynamics 34,* 313–330.

Wegner, D.M. (2002) *The Illusion of Conscious Will.* Cambridge, MA: MIT Press.

Williams, K.D. (2001) *Ostracism. The Power of Silence.* London: The Guilford Press.

Woods, M. (2011) 'An ethic of care in nursing: Past, present and future considerations.' *Ethics and Social Welfare 5,* 3, 266–276.

Zerubavel, E. (2006) *The Elephant in the Room: Silence and Denial in Everyday Life.* Oxford: Oxford University Press.

Zimbardo, P. (2008) 'The Psychology of Evil.' *TED Talk.* Accessed on 14 November 2014 from www.ted.com/talks/philip_zimbardo_on_the_psychology_of_evil.

Zipparo, L. (1999) 'Encouraging public sector employees to report workplace corruption.' *Australian Journal of Public Administration 5,* 2, 83–93.

SUBJECT INDEX

AUTHOR INDEX